SHIATSU
FOR TWO

SHIATSU FOR TWO

A Manual for Beginners

Hajo Hadeler

Harbour Publishing Co. Ltd.
1988

Text © Hajo Hadeler 1988
Illustrations © Gaye Hammond 1988
Cover and Book Design by Gaye Hammond
ISBN 0-920080-92-8

Harbour Publishing Co. Ltd.
Box 219, Madeira Park, B.C.
Canada   V0N 2H0

Canadian Cataloguing in Publication Data

Hadeler, Hajo, 1931-
Shiatsu for two

ISBN 0-920080-92-8

1.   Acupressure.   I.   Title.
RM723.A27H33   1988   615.8'22   C88-091190-5

Printed in Canada by Friesen Printers

None of this would have happened without the infinite patience of my excellent teachers—

Wanchai Arthavedvoravudhi, Bangkok, Thailand
Habran Singh, Sarnath, India
One Sun, Sunim, Korea and Steveston, B.C.

I am grateful.

        hh

TABLE OF CONTENTS

FOREWORD

Shiatsu is neither occult nor mythical. It merely has very ancient roots in the area along the Yellow River. It is based on several thousand years of Chinese medicine, the longest uninterrupted development of medical science we have on the planet. History has shown that Chinese medicine was, and is, quite capable of looking after the therapeutic needs of what has become the most populous country on earth.

Today, Shiatsu is far and away the least expensive method of preventive medicine, drug-free and with no adverse side-effects.

The partner method shown in this book is based on meridional therapy, which goes back to the ancient Chinese system of Acupuncture and beyond that to the Ayurveda of India. Yoga and Shiatsu have much in common. Emphasis is placed on purification and detoxification of the entire body—holistic preventive medicine—rather than on momentary pain relief through treatment of one or more of the several hundred pressure points. Uncertainty about the precise location of these tsubos restrains many people from giving Shiatsu to someone in need. On the other hand, encyclopedic knowledge of every single pressure point may turn Shiatsu into mere push-button quackery, which it was never meant to be (push here and your haemorrhoids will go away, push there and the ringing in your ears will stop, push another place and your asthma of five years vanishes).

Not only is meridional therapy easier to learn: the beneficial effects for the two people involved are lasting and reach far beyond physical well-being.

He and she are used interchangeably in the text, of course.

THIS YOU SHOULD KNOW

BACKGROUND

The Japanese word SHI-ATSU means finger pressure. Shiatsu is one of a number of systems of healing where finger pressure is applied to the human body along normally invisible lines, and at certain spots which are also not normally visible. The system is derived from Chinese Acupuncture. It uses the same pathways of energy, the meridians, and the same points, the tsubos. The essential difference is that, unlike an Acupuncturist, a Shiatsu practitioner uses no needles.

Shiatsu is an energetic system of healing. It balances the body's energy field by removing blockages in the pathways and by guiding surplus energy into depleted areas. The pathways were found by careful observation and have been known for several thousand years. Knowledge of these energy paths can be traced from Japan via Korea back to China, and from there to India and the Ayurveda, the ancient Hindu art of medicine and prolonging life.

SHIATSU AS PREVENTION

Shiatsu is priceless as preventive medicine, as a system that deals effectively with the daily disturbances to our health and well-being which show up as fatigue, headache, shortness of breath, lower back pain, constipation, heartburn and a hundred other red warning lights that tell us: all is not well. We are not sick enough to see a doctor, yet we are not healthy either, so we muddle through, as most people on this planet do.

Left untreated for years, small complaints have the annoying habit of turning into chronic complaints. Disturbance has become destruction—and that is one reason

3

ANCIENT AND MODERN HEALING SYSTEMS

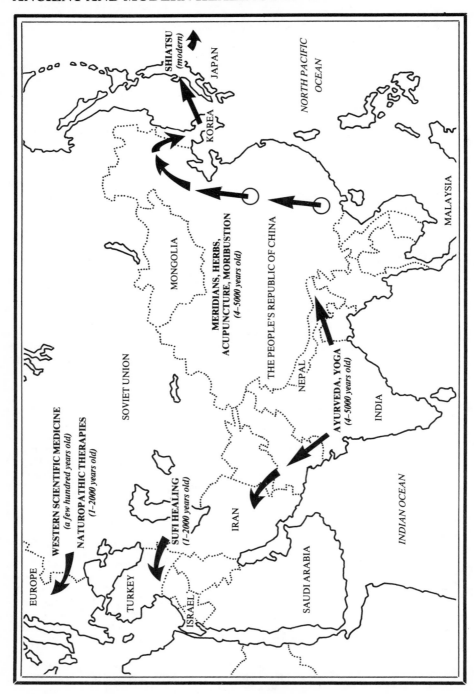

why the cost of health is skyrocketing today. Chronic diseases are on the increase. Once destruction has begun, Shiatsu can only alleviate the symptoms. It has limits; it is not effective against mental diseases, psychological disorders, deficiency and hereditary diseases, cancer, advanced infectious diseases, advanced cirrhosis of the liver and other forms of destruction. In cases like these, it is valuable as an additional, non-poisonous, drug-free therapy.

While it is reassuring to know that you can do no harm, Shiatsu does not produce miracles overnight. It encourages the body to heal itself, but complete restoration of perfect health is rarely ever possible after destruction has begun. Rather: start practicing Shiatsu early in life and regularly, catch disturbances before they can cause permanent damage, and thus stay as healthy as you can be at all times.

EAST VS WEST

Chinese doctors, it is said, were only paid as long as their patients remained healthy. Once disease set in, no more money changed hands and the reputation of the healer dropped like a stone in a pond. This is why Oriental medicine developed an elaborate system of diagnosis, detective work in the grey area between minor complaint and full-blown disease. Nothing was overlooked. Shortness of breath was treated before it became chronic asthma. Heartburn was treated before it turned into chronic gastritis. Cold feet were treated before poor peripheral circulation led to a breakdown of the cardiovascular system. Buzzing in the ears was treated before it turned into high-pitched ringing, tinnitus, which is difficult to cure and may signal the beginning of total hearing loss.

Regular house calls kept an Oriental healer abreast of early symptoms, and he was particularly aware of stressful situations in his patient's life which, scientific medicine has shown, alter stress hormone levels. These hormones (ACTH, cortisone and others) prepare the human body for action, but altered levels also suppress immune responses and thus open the doors for virus and bacterial attacks.

Few Western doctors make house calls today, and the grey area of early symptoms is largely ignored by both doctor and patient. If the symptoms are bothersome and interfere with daily life and all-important work, they are suppressed. Case in point: the shelves filled with cold remedies in my neighborhood drugstore are fifteen feet long. None of these potions, capsules and pills cures a cold, but they will stop your nose from running, your eyes from watering, and they will cause you not to sneeze, so that you can "get on with the job." Instead of assisting your body to fight the virus, these drugs incarcerate the body's police and the culprits have free rein.

Oriental medicine doesn't work that way. Symptoms are not

masked or disguised. Pseudo-health is not acceptable. As a first step, everything will be done to help your body fight the current infection—and it is the whole body that is involved, not just the mucous membrane of your nose; holistic health, instead of the ear-nose-throat specialist of scientific medicine. The cold shouldn't have happened in the first place, but since it did—what caused the weakness in your immune system? Why did your body permit the virus to find a host cell? The logical next step, then, is to strengthen your body, so that it can guard against future virus attacks.

It is an unending task. The key is regularity: to keep the energy household of the human body in perfect balance at all times, so that it can help itself and cure itself, something it does remarkably well most of the time, but not always. Regular Shiatsu keeps the energy household balanced.

THIS BOOK

We want to do something for our health, but instead of keeping healthy, we keep fit, which is not the same thing. We bounce around to loud, rhythmic music and do aerobics. We earnestly push weights, develop muscles, ride exercise bicycles that go nowhere, and jog around the block. In our pursuit of excellence we are fit and fatigued, well-muscled and sick, tanned and depressed.

Few of us are lucky enough to have a Shiatsu practitioner come around once or twice a month, use pulse diagnosis to check us out and then work for a while on two or more of the indicated meridians until YIN and YANG, the two components of our life energy, CHI, are in perfect balance again. There are simply not enough Shiatsu practitioners around.

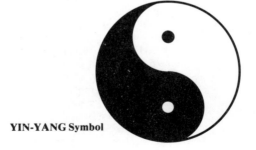

YIN-YANG Symbol

Hence this book: to show you a system which, applied slowly and with loving concern in a restful setting, will take care of your everyday aches and pains by restoring the energy balance of your body to perfection. Regular Shiatsu, even by an inexperienced practitioner, tends to catch disturbances well before they turn into destruction. Shiatsu will keep you as healthy as you can be. Colds become less frequent. Menstrual disorders, headaches, rheumatic and arthritic pain will be alleviated and may disappear altogether with regular Shiatsu.

SHIATSU FOR TWO

While not impossible to do it alone, it has been my experience that Shiatsu is best practiced with a friend. For one, it is difficult to reach and follow some of the meridians conveniently around the entire body. On a higher level, it is important to break out of the narcissistic shell that traps many students into an egocentric pattern of thinking. "I want to be healthy! I have stomach pains. I...I...I...!" Shiatsu at its very best is an interpersonal happening: two people who care for each other work together in such a way that they touch on a level far deeper than the mere physical. To use a Yoga expression: the energy fields (subtle bodies) of both partners should blend. There can be no walls between giver and receiver. Ultimately, both will benefit. There is nothing mystic or occult about this. Lovers holding hands surely experience more than mere touch.

As male-female relationships develop, links beyond simple physical attraction are discovered. Finding out how and where your partner hides accumulated daily stresses can be amusing.

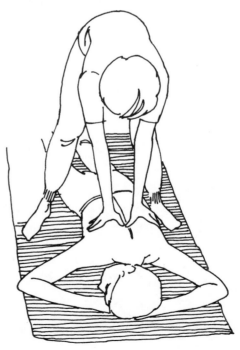

Getting rid of them is joy! Learning to understand and help on this level will make any relationship more authentic and lessen the chances of game-playing and manipulation. Naturally, all that is said applies to male-male and female-female relationships as well. The aim is helping each other along the way to glowing, beautiful health—both physical and mental. As you are aware, the two can not be separated. And what is life without health?

MERIDIANS

BACKGROUND

Even though it is today an accepted term among Shiatsu practitioners and lay persons alike, meridian is an unfortunate choice of word. It conjures up images of artificial geographical lines running in great circles over both poles and dividing our planet into orange slices. Meridians in Shiatsu don't do that. It would be more helpful to think of them as open pathways or channels along which the energy of life surges in greater concentration, and more accessibly, than elsewhere in the body.

Western scientific medicine has so far been unable to prove the existence of energetic channels in the human body. The system works, yet no specific organ or substrate has been found that transports the energy of life in a manner similar to the way information is passed along the nervous system from one neuron to another, for example, or the way blood circulates through veins and arteries.

Some European researchers think that the energy in Shiatsu and Acupuncture meridians uses pathways that already exist as receptor chains in well-known regulatory mechanisms. The flight-or-fight response, for example, activates the entire sympathetic nervous system and stimulates cortisol release, which in turn regulates the body's metabolism so that it can deal with a stressful situation. Messages race back and forth between the hypothalamus, receptors of the body, and virtually all areas of the brain. These same pathways could double as channels for the energy of life when survival is not threatened. (Dr. Kim Bongham of Pyongyang University, North Korea, claimed to have found a histological substrate for the energy pathways, but other researchers have so far been unable to locate his Kyungrak System again.)

YIN, YANG AND CHI

The energy we are dealing with is called CHI in Chinese. Literally translated, this means breath, breath of life. Its two components are YANG and YIN. If you think of them in terms of positive and negative, black and white, hot and cold, heaven and earth, man and woman, surplus and need, you are on the right track. One can not exist without the other. Without white, we have no way of knowing what black is. Without hot there can be no cold. If you connect a light bulb to only one pole of your car's battery, the bulb will not light up—it needs the other pole to work.

This thinking in terms of complementary dualism rather than conflict has remained strong throughout Chinese history and is reflected in art, poetry, architecture and everyday life. YANG and YIN, in harmonious balance, make up CHI, the universal energy, which maintains creation the way we perceive it. Our bodies reflect this harmony. If they don't, we are not well and need help.

Over thousands of years of patient observation, the Chinese have found twelve major YIN-YANG meridians and a number of minor ones in the human body. The major meridians and two special vessels concern us in this book.

YIN and YANG are complementary forces rather than absolutes. They are in a constant state of flux. Here are some examples:

YIN	YANG
female	male
wet	dry
negative	positive
vegetable	animal
universal	specific
passive	active
cold	hot
dark	bright
soft	hard
humid climate	dry climate
defensive	aggressive
future-oriented	past-oriented
spiritual	material
fragile	tough

MERIDIANS

Heart	Small Intestine
Kidney	Urinary Bladder
Heart Constrictor	Triple Heater
Liver	Gallbladder
Lung	Large Intestine
Spleen-Pancreas	Stomach

THE MERIDIANS

The six YANG meridians run from heaven to earth, the six YIN meridians run from earth to heaven. Each meridian exists as part of a YIN-YANG pair. Thus, the Urinary Bladder meridian (YANG) has a partner in the Kidney meridian (YIN), while the Lung meridian (YIN) has the Large Intestine meridian (YANG) for a partner. Each meridian also exists as a mirror image of itself. This means that the Kidney meridian on the right side of your body has a mirror image on the left side. It is important to remember that this is not a YIN-YANG pair. The Kidney meridian is always YIN, whether it is on the left or right side of the body. When we talk about the Kidney meridian, we mean the pair, and it always starts under your feet and the energy flow is upwards, from Earth to Heaven, in true YIN fashion.

The table (below) shows all twelve meridians in the classical Chinese order, which starts with the Heart meridian as number one. The column on the right indicates the ideal time for most effective work on the given meridian. Since it may not always be possible to observe this, keep in mind that few practitioners ever work under perfect time conditions, yet patients are cured all the same.

1	Heart	H	YIN	12–2 p.m.
2	Small Intestine	SI	YANG	2–4 p.m.
3	Urinary Bladder	UB	YANG	4–6 p.m.
4	Kidney	KI	YIN	6–8 p.m.
5	Heart Constrictor	HC	YIN	8–10 p.m.
6	Triple Heater	TH	YANG	10–12 p.m.
7	Gallbladder	GB	YANG	12–2 a.m.
8	Liver	LV	YIN	2–4 a.m.
9	Lung	LU	YIN	4–6 a.m.
10	Large Intestine	LI	YANG	6–8 a.m.
11	Stomach	ST	YANG	8–10 a.m.
12	Spleen–Pancreas	SP	YIN	10–12 a.m.

The two additional energy channels are called Governor vessel (GV) and Conception vessel (CV).

As you can see, the table is divided into three sections of four meridians. Each group of four represents one cycle of energy, and in all three cycles the energy flows in a similar pattern.

The first cycle starts with the Heart meridian (H). This YIN meridian follows the inside of the upper arm, goes down the inside of the forearm and runs along the wrist joint. It ends approximately an eighth of an inch from the inside corner of the nail on the little finger. Now it turns YANG (SI) and marches up the outside of the arm to the shoulder, where it zig-zags, runs along the neck to the cheek and ends in front of the ear. From the skull the energy flow continues downward in two channels on either side of the spine in the Urinary Bladder meridian (UB), still YANG, ends at the little toe, turns YIN, and flows up again in the Kidney meridian (KI), which ends where the clavicle meets the sternum.

A few things must be pointed out here. First, the Heart meridian is YIN (Earth to Heaven), and yet we describe the energy flow as moving downward. This is because, during treatment, your partner is either sitting down or lying on his back, with both arms comfortably placed on either side of the trunk, fingers pointing toward the feet, i.e. down. The position in which the ancient Chinese saw a healthy human being was different: he was standing up, feet slightly apart, both arms raised and stretched toward heaven, palms up and the head tilted backwards. Now the energy in the Heart meridian flows up, from Earth to Heaven—YIN.

The pattern of energy in every cycle is YIN-YANG-YANG-YIN and we can say that some meridians run nearly parallel to each other over long distances—nearly, but not quite.

Every cycle begins at the chest, moves up the arm (YIN) to a finger, down the arm (YANG) to the head, down the trunk (YANG) to a toe and back up (YIN) to the chest.

It is worth noting that all YIN meridians run along the inside of arms and legs—YIN...in. YANG meridians continue along the outside, but no mnemonic device offers itself to remember this. About 365 pressure points or tsubos are located along the meridians. The diameter of a tsubo is usually less than that of an ordinary lead pencil (1/8 to 1/16 of an inch), and even under the best of circumstances they are much more difficult to find than the dark spots on a crimson ladybug.

LOCATING MERIDIANS

On Sun, Sunim, one of my teachers, is a Buddhist monk and his head is shaven. He carefully pulled out one of my hairs and sealed it in a plain envelope. Handing it to me, he said, "Find, please!" This taught me that the tip of my middle finger is about twice as sensitive to minute bulges as any of the other fingers. Try it!

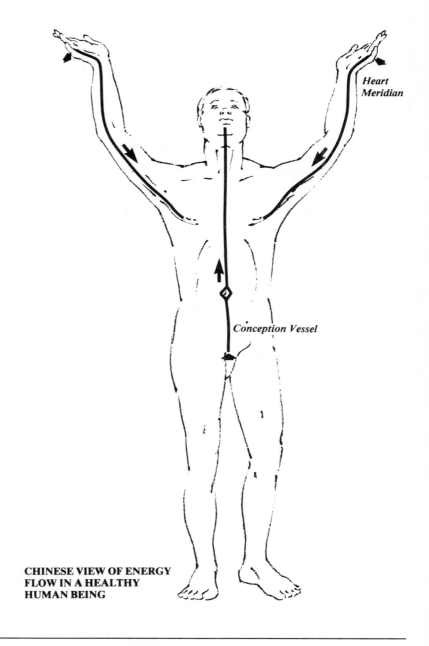

Heart Meridian

Conception Vessel

**CHINESE VIEW OF ENERGY
FLOW IN A HEALTHY
HUMAN BEING**

Most tsubos are more difficult to find than a hair in an envelope. As human beings we are all recognizably built from roughly the same blueprint, but the key word is roughly: individual differences account for the fact that no two tsubos

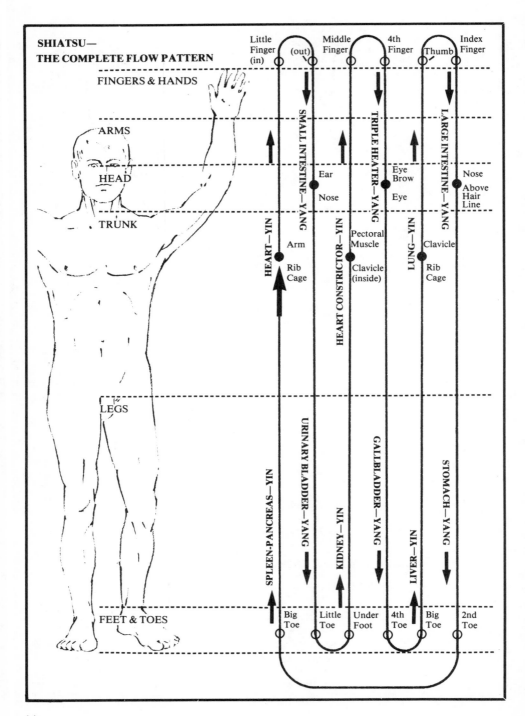

SHIATSU—
THE COMPLETE FLOW PATTERN

FINGERS & HANDS

ARMS

HEAD

TRUNK

LEGS

FEET & TOES

Little Finger (in)   (out)   Middle Finger   4th Finger   Thumb   Index Finger

SMALL INTESTINE—YANG

Ear
Nose

HEART—YIN

Arm
Rib Cage

TRIPLE HEATER—YANG

Eye Brow
Eye

HEART CONSTRICTOR—YIN

Pectoral Muscle
Clavicle (inside)

LARGE INTESTINE—YANG

Nose
Above Hair Line

LUNG—YIN

Clavicle
Rib Cage

SPLEEN-PANCREAS—YIN

URINARY BLADDER—YANG

KIDNEY—YIN

GALLBLADDER—YANG

LIVER—YIN

STOMACH—YANG

Big Toe   Little Toe   Under Foot   4th Toe   Big Toe   2nd Toe

are ever in exactly the same location on two people. Worse yet, as your physical condition and your mood change from day to day and from hour to hour, so, minutely, does the location of a given pressure point change.

This is why many people fail to find relief, even though they have bought a beautifully illustrated pressure point atlas and stab their finger tips at all the indicated points. It isn't quite that simple.

To a lesser degree, what has been said about the tsubos also applies to the meridians: no two people have them in exactly the same place. However, the body under your fingers is full of bumps and hollows. The knuckles protruding from the spine can be counted. Hard and soft muscles form distinct patterns under the skin and the skeleton provides a framework of bones and joints. These are all reliable topographic features that give you beacons and sign posts to help you establish the course of a meridian.

At this time in your endeavour it is much more important to learn the road map of meridians on the surface of your partner's body, than to worry about finding individual tsubos. Inevitably, you will touch a few by luck and accident. As time goes on, you will find more. But it is not wise for a beginner to rely on an ability that has yet to be developed. Before such happy accidents will happen consistently and become your certain knowledge, the road maps of energy will have to be learned. Seldom can it be done without the cooperation of your partner, who has to tell you if touching a certain spot feels different to her. This response will guide you until you have developed the ability, a combination of touch and intuition, love, care and being in tune, a sensation unlike any other.

There is no easy way to teach your fingers a path that they will then remember forever. Nobody can do this for you. The basic training of a professional Shiatsu practitioner in Korea takes six years, but even after that the learning never stops. You will make your own discoveries about the mysteries of the human body as people come and ask you for help. You will find that what works in one person may not work in another. No two headaches are exactly the same, and lower back aches will test your understanding of YIN-YANG patterns to the limit.

For the time being it is best to set all expectations about healing aside. This way you will not be disappointed if your partner does not get well instantly. Expect nothing. Inevitably there will be small successes and they will light your path like candles. Treasure them. They are precious. In time there will be many.

If there is no healing for a long while, don't be discouraged. Other, equally important things are occurring. If you set aside an evening every week to practice Shiatsu with your partner, the relationship is bound to deepen and blossom. You will grow together as you discover not just meridians, but each other.

15

ROAD MAPS OF ENERGY

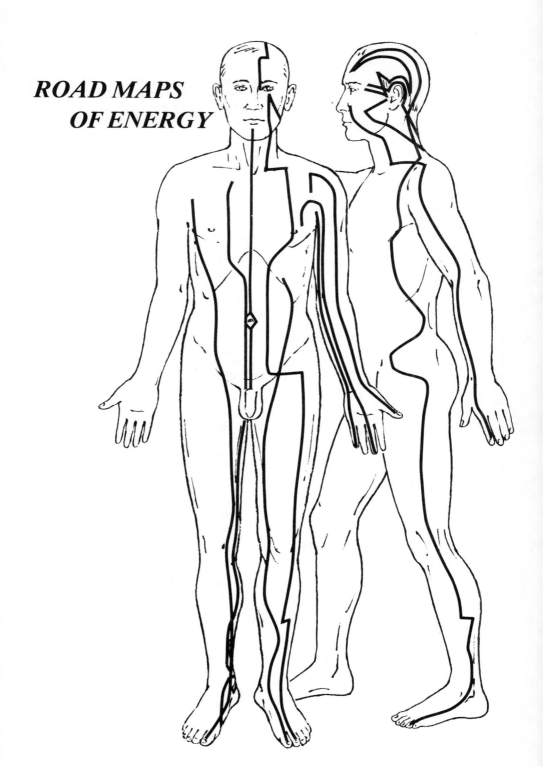

1. HEART – (H) – Yin

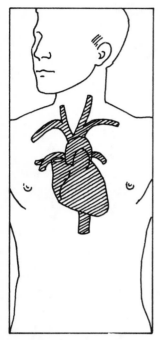

The heart is two pumps in one assembly of cardiac muscle, located in the chest cavity to the left of centre. Slightly larger than your fist, the heart has an intricate system of valves to prevent the back flow of blood. Every contraction of the muscle sends a stream of blood through the aorta into the arteries. From there it flows through arterioles and tiny capillaries into the veins and back to the heart, only to be sent through another chamber and out the pulmonary artery into the lungs, where carbon dioxide is eliminated and oxygen is loaded. Then the cycle starts again.

The English physician William Harvey demonstrated this in 1628, and Western medicine reckons the beginning of Experimental Physiology from this year. Like gun powder, rockets, compass and printing press, the cardiovascular cycle was known in China long before the time of Harvey, and Acupuncture was already more than four thousand years old.

Oriental medicine counts the heart among the five essential organs of the human body. West and East meet in their popular view that the heart is more than merely a pump; the psychic connection is understood when we use phrases like heart and soul, to take heart, his heart was in his mouth, after my own heart and heart-rending. The heart is seen as the seat of the affections, of courage, will and love. It should not surprise us, therefore, that the Heart meridian in Shiatsu also functions as governor of spirit and emotions.

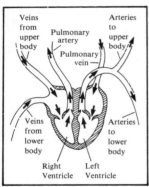

Veins from upper body	Pulmonary artery		Arteries to upper body
Pulmonary vein			
Veins from lower body			Arteries to lower body
	Right Ventricle	Left Ventricle	

Flow of Blood

Location The Heart meridian (YIN...in) begins on the rib cage close to the arm pit. From there it runs along the biceps to a point on the elbow. This waypoint is easy to find. Bend the arm and a fold appears inside the elbow. The meridian passes over the inside end of the fold and continues along forearm, wrist and palm, and ends on the inside of the little finger very close to the inside base of the nail.

Function Beyond balancing the cardiovascular cycle, treating the Heart meridian will prove effective against such problems as stage fright or anxiety before an examination, and such symptoms as nervous tension, poor appetite, restlessness, sweaty palms and excessive underarm odour. If you examine these symptoms, you will find that all are related to unrelieved stress.

Treatment There is no best position for treating the Heart meridian. It is easily accessible whether the receiver is sitting down or lying on his back, as long as the arm remains relaxed.

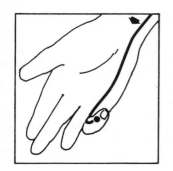

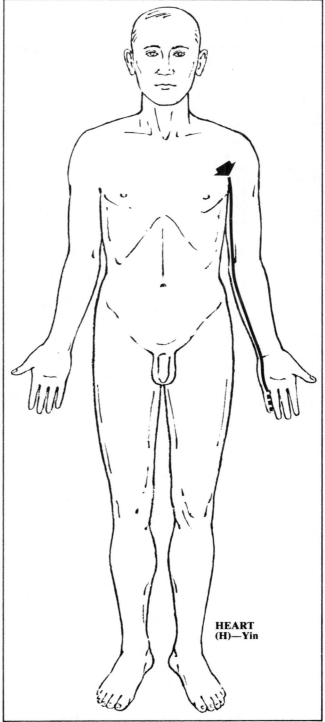

**HEART
(H)—Yin**

2. SMALL INTESTINE – (SI) – Yang

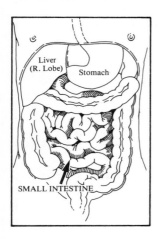

Liver
(R. Lobe) Stomach

SMALL INTESTINE

Before the food we eat can do us any good, it must be broken down into molecules of a size that can be absorbed through the cell walls of the gastrointestinal tract. The breaking down is called digestion. It starts in the mouth and ends when the remaining waste is eliminated from the body.

Nearly all of the substances we eat are digested and absorbed in the small intestine, which is a coiled tube that connects the stomach with the large intestine. The tube is about nine feet long and has a diameter of 1½ inches. The section closest to the stomach is called the duodenum, Latin for twelve, because it is the length of twelve fingers placed side by side (about 8 inches). Next follows the jejunum and finally the longest segment, the ileum.

Except, perhaps, for the sense of hearing, all other senses are actively involved when we eat. Even emotional states come into play: anticipation may cause us to salivate like Pavlov's dog. Sight, smell, taste and touch activate neurons which in turn stimulate cells to secrete anything from acid to hormones to pepsinogen, the inactive form of pepsin, an enzyme that helps to split proteins into amino acids.

Digestion is a complex matter. Any malfunction in the system will affect the entire body either through lack of nutrition or through an imbalance in the salt and water household. Oriental and Western medicine essentially hold the same views.

Location The meridian associated with the Small Intestine (SI) receives its energy from the Heart meridian (H), which ends close to the inside base of the nail of the little finger. As a YANG meridian, SI begins near the outside base of the same fingernail and ends in front and close to the centre of the ear. It runs along the outside of palm and wrist, past the elbow and up to the shoulder—note the V in its path—then up to the neck, which has been marked as a point of interest: SI crosses paths with TH and G here, and the LI meridian passes very close. (More about this interesting region in the chapter on treatment.) SI continues across the jawbone to a point under the cheekbone and in line with the outer corner of the eye. It ends near the ear.

Function Mucus is secreted along the entire length of the gastrointestinal tract. This is necessary for lubrication as well as for protection of the sensitive inner surface from acids, digesting enzymes and bile salts. Treating the Small Intestine meridian has a particularly beneficial effect on all mucus-related problems in the human body. This includes diseases like sty and conjunctivitis (eye) as well as rhinitis (hay fever), vaginitis and generally all inflammations of mucous membranes that produce catarrhal symptoms, e.g. a watery discharge. In addition, regular treatment of SI is effective against poor digestion and constipation as well as irregularities in the menstrual cycle.

Treatment Since SI involves arm, shoulder and head, it should be treated with the receiver lying down.

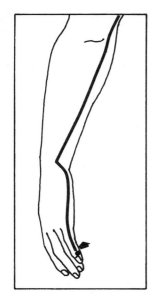

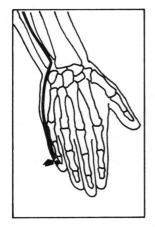

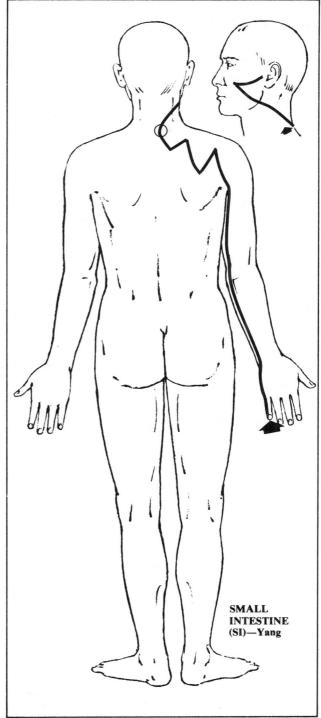

**SMALL
INTESTINE
(SI)—Yang**

3. URINARY BLADDER – (UB) – Yang

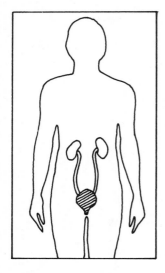

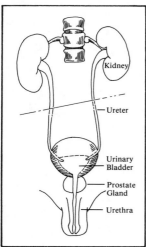

Kidney

Ureter

Urinary Bladder

Prostate Gland

Urethra

Such a small organ, the urinary bladder, yet in Oriental medicine it connects with the longest of all twelve major meridians. The urinary bladder is no more than a holding tank. It stores the urine, which is produced in the kidneys and conveyed to the bladder via the two ureters. The bladder is drained by the urethra, which in males is about 8 inches long, compared with 1 ½ inches in females.

The teachings of ancient Oriental medicine essentially correspond to these findings of Western science, with the additional belief that fluids left over in the small intestine after digestion of solid food are thought to drain through the intestinal wall and accumulate in the bladder as well. The idea is not entirely without merit if we consider that a steak, for example, comprises up to 70 percent water.

What makes UB especially interesting for the Shiatsu practitioner is the fact that diagnostic points for each of the twelve major meridians can be found on its first branch down the back. More about this in the chapter on diagnosis.

Location The Urinary Bladder meridian governs elimination, purification and detoxification in the human body. It begins on either side of the nose, just above the points where your sunglasses rest. YANG meridians normally run from heaven to earth, from the highest point down to the feet. Please recall the ancient Chinese view of a healthy human being: erect, arms raised, palms up and head tilted backwards. This position brings the beginning of UB to the highest point of the head (see page 13).

From the nose, the meridian continues over the head, approximately two fingerbreadths from either side of the centre line, and runs down either side of the spine to the buttocks—note the jog—then it continues down the back of upper and lower leg and along the outside of the foot and ends within 1/16 inch of the nail on the little toe. This is the first branch.

The second branch starts below the back of the head and continues down the back at a distance of two fingerbreadths outside the first branch. (When you measure this, use your receiver's fingers: they are in proportion.) Both branches join below the buttocks and continue as one to the little toe.

Function As you can see from the drawings, UB courses from the head down through the entire posterior or dorsal landscape of the human body. Shiatsu treatment of UB in the head region reduces headaches and alleviates the symptoms of conjunctivitis and sinusitis as well as inflammation in the nose area. Point massage along the upper back down to the tips of the shoulder blades eases bronchitis, coughing and bronchial asthma. Treatment of middle and lower back relieves liver complaints as well as stomach cramps and digestive disorders, e.g. both constipation and diarrhea. It has also proven effective against general fatigue, pain caused by rheumatic diseases, and lumbago. The second branch of UB in this region affects chronic skin diseases.

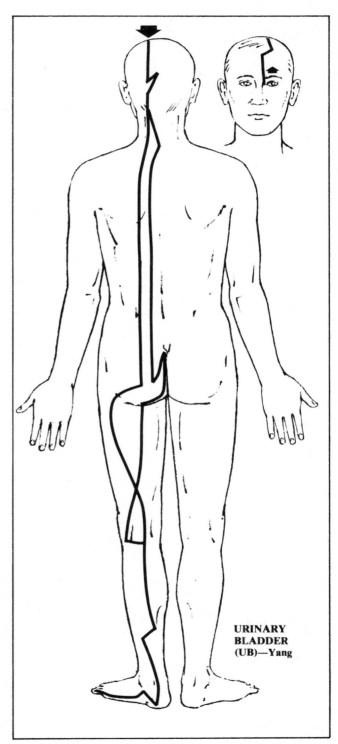

**URINARY
BLADDER
(UB)—Yang**

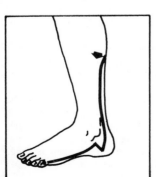

23

UB therapy of upper and lower leg is very useful against abnormalities of the metabolism and has a calming and normalizing effect on all chemical reactions taking place in the body. Finally, Shiatsu treatment of the feet can be most effective against any kind of pain anywhere in the body, from sore muscles and sciatic complaints to headaches and painful cramps. Point massage here also alleviates insomnia and induces sleep.

Treatment Even though UB is the longest of all the major meridians, its route is not particularly difficult to remember. The head is best treated while your partner is sitting up, one side at a time, using your free hand for support and assurance. Once you are ready to work on neck, trunk and legs, your receiver should rest face-down on the carpet with a small pillow for head support. Work on both inner branches at the same time, then both outer branches. To do this, you can either straddle your receiver, or you can kneel alongside. Then work on one leg at a time. The order is not important, but once you have reached the inside of the knee it is best to support the lower leg by kneeling down and placing the foot of your partner across your thigh. That way, the remainder of the meridian is easily accessible right down to the little toe. Treat the other leg the same way and return it gently to the carpet. Don't let your partner do that!

4. KIDNEY – (KI) – Yin

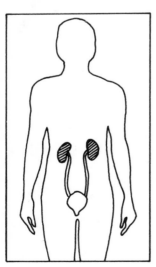

We have two kidneys. They are located near the back of the body on either side of the spine, roughly in the mid-section. The popular concept of their function is that they are garbage disposal units, but this is only half the story. The more important but lesser known half is their regulation of sodium, water, potassium, calcium, magnesium, sulphate, phosphate and hydrogen ion concentrations in the body—and this is only a partial list. The regulatory process is so finely tuned that what is excreted one moment may be retained the next, because the balance has shifted in the body. Some of this recent Western knowledge reflects the teachings of ancient Oriental medicine, which viewed the kidney as one of the five essential organs. Its role in detoxification and purification was understood and the kidneys were said to achieve control over mental stress by regulating hormone secretion.

Location The meridian begins under your foot between the balls of the big and little toes. Since it is a YIN meridian, the path of energy moves to the inside of the leg and upwards past the knee to the groin. From there it runs less than one inch from either side of the navel and up to the rib cage, where it ends near the lowest point of the clavicles.

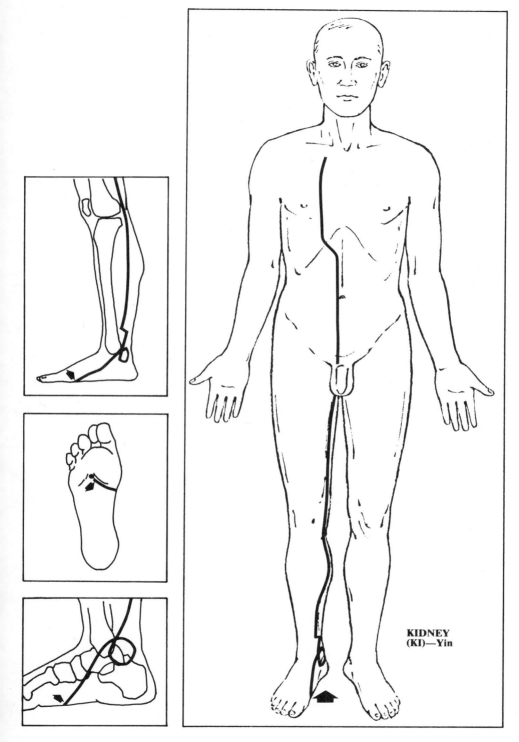

**KIDNEY
(KI)—Yin**

25

KIDNEY – (KI) – YIN, CONT'D

Function Working on the Kidney meridian normalizes the many regulatory functions of the kidney. The resulting improved hormonal balance causes general fatigue to disappear, along with menstrual irregularities, fear, sadness, indecision, some forms of migraine headache and also asthma—the kind that becomes worse when the weather is cold and wet.

Treatment Since the Kidney meridian runs on the ventral side of the body, your partner must turn over and rest on his back. Treat each leg separately up to the groin. Support the leg with your free hand as you do this. From the groin up to the end of the meridian, straddle your partner and work on both sides of the body at once.

KI completes the first YIN-YANG-YANG-YIN cycle.

5. HEART CONSTRICTOR – (HC) – Yin

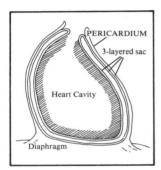

The French name for this meridian is Maitre du coeur—Master of the Heart. It fits better than Heart Constrictor, because there is nothing constricting about this meridian in the sense that it squeezes or condenses an organ and thus hinders its movements. We are talking about the pericardium, the membranous sac that surrounds the heart. Oriental medicine does not regard it as an isolated organ, because its function is to serve the heart. It acts as Prime Minister in a country where the heart is the Emperor. Its role can not be separated from that of the heart. An indication of its effectiveness is provided in another name it carries: the meridian for circulation and sex.

Location HC is a YIN meridian that begins one finger-breadth outside the nipples, curves around the armpit, then follows a course along the inside of the upper arm along the biceps and to the elbow. Now it subtly changes into the centre lane of the inner forearm and heads straight for a line in the hand that palmists call the Line of Fate. This line is followed to the root of the middle finger. Then HC swings around to the thumb side of the middle finger and ends approximately 1/8 inch from the base of the fingernail.

Function As may be expected from its close association with the heart, treating HC supplements treatment of the Heart meridian and normalizes variances in the cardiovascular system. Circulation, hormonal balance and sexual dysfunction also benefit from regular Shiatsu on this meridian. One of the pressure points on HC was the major tsubo for the treatment of malaria in ancient China (HC 6).

Treatment HC can be treated with the receiver lying down or sitting up. If you have completed KI, why not continue with HC?

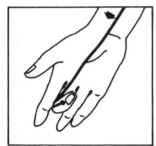

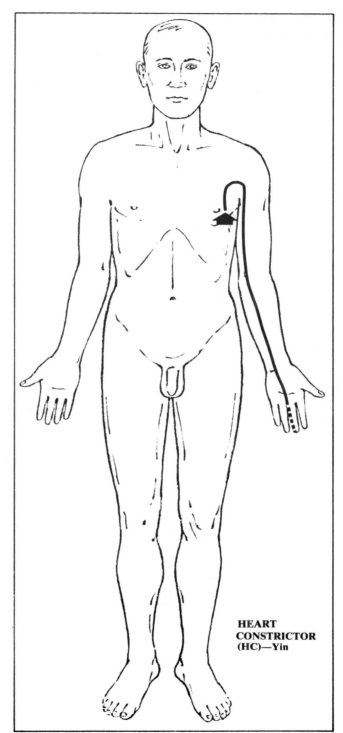

**HEART
CONSTRICTOR
(HC)—Yin**

6. TRIPLE HEATER – (TH) – Yang

When a child is conceived, the life energy from both parents finds a new vessel in which to merge, and a new being develops. Until birth, all the energies the child receives are filtered through the mother's body. This is a protective preparation for the day of birth, when the child has to mobilize its own equipment to deal with the many forms of energy life offers. A pat on the behind shocks the respiratory apparatus into audible activity. Mother's milk impels the digestive tract to function. The skin is open to touch, sun, wind and rain, the ears receive messages, and all that energy has to be processed.

Location   The entity that does the processing is the Triple Heater (TH). Western medicine has no equivalent for this Oriental conception, and no organ is attached to the name. If you think of heat as converted energy, then the meaning is easier to comprehend. The meridian starts close to the nail on the ring finger and moves along the back of the hand, up the back of the forearm and upper arm to the middle of the shoulder, then along the side of the neck up to the mastoid process. It closely circles the ear and ends near the outer part of the eyebrow.

Function   Functionally, TH is concerned with respiration, digestion and the urogenital tract—one heater for each, hence the threefold heater. Since any disturbance in these areas inevitably affects the whole body, treating TH improves the entire constitution. It should always be used when the receiver is recovering from a major illness. Acupuncturists know that the primary point against rheumatic complaints can be found on this meridian (TH 6). Other important points on TH are helpful against facial neuralgias and those that affect shoulder and neck. In all, TH is an excellent energy channel to work on for toning and general well-being.

Treatment   TH is easy to reach with the receiver sitting up or lying down.

7. GALLBLADDER – (GB) – Yang

The gallbladder is shaped like a small pear and has its own little niche on the underside of the liver. It is a storage sac that holds about 1/3 cup of bile. The bile is produced in the liver and sent from there to the duodenum. When the duodenum does not need any more bile, a sphincter muscle closes and the bile has no place to go but into the gallbladder, where it is saved for future use. When next you eat, the sphincter muscle relaxes and bile flows into the duodenum again.

Between meals the bile in the gallbladder is concentrated and acidified into a potent mix. It holds bile salts, which help

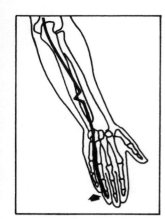

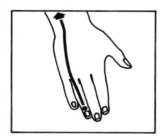

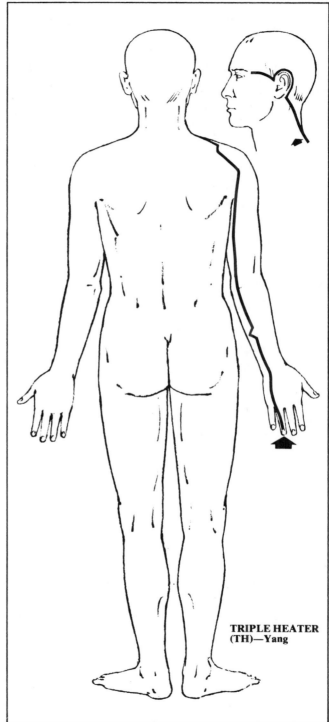

**TRIPLE HEATER
(TH)—Yang**

GALLBLADDER – (GB) – YANG, CONT'D

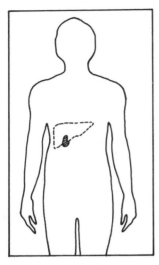

Front View

Liver

Stomach

GALLBLADDER

Back View

Liver

GALLBLADDER

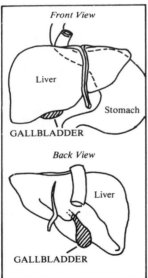

digest fat. It also contains pigments, cholesterol, lecithin and trace metals. Both Western medicine and Oriental healing concur in their assessments of the organ.

Location   The Gallbladder meridian covers the body from head to toe. As a YANG meridian it runs along the outside of the extremities and down. Its path begins with a nearly straight line from the outer corner of the eye to the ear. It zig-zags and curls around the ear and comes to a point two fingerbreadths above the eyebrows and in line with the pupils. From here it goes up to the hairline, across the head and down to a point on top of the shoulder. Then it moves along the side of the body in three curves and comes to rest where the big thighbone can be felt in the hip. Now it continues as a large centre channel down the outside of the leg and proceeds forward of the outer ankle, then curves with the foot and ends near the outside base of the nail on the fourth toe.

Function   Since the meridian covers so much territory, treatment can be expected to affect many regions of the body. Carefully working along GB on the head relieves symptoms connected with eye diseases, especially conjunctivitis, but also migraine headaches that are caused by eye disorders. Neuralgias, i.e. pain of the facial nerves, are also alleviated.

Regular treatment of GB along the trunk effectively normalizes not only disorders of the gallbladder itself, biliary colic for example, but also liver ailments and diseases connected with poor digestion of fats, which may show up as obesity in spite of low fat consumption. Shiatsu will not dissolve gallstones, but lumbago and sciatica benefit and the symptoms of hormonal imbalance tend to disappear, especially if they show up as skin rash. Along the lower leg, GB treatment benefits muscular paresis (where motion is affected, but not sensation) and diseases of all joints, particularly the large ones like hip, shoulder and knee.

Treatment   The head portion of GB is best treated with the receiver sitting up. Start by doing one side of the head at a time and use the free hand for support. In order to do the lateral run of GB, the receiver is best placed on the carpet again, with a pillow for head support. It does not matter whether the leg is bent or straight, but it is important that your partner be as comfortable as possible and that there is little or no muscular tension in the leg.

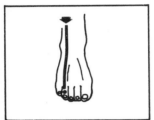

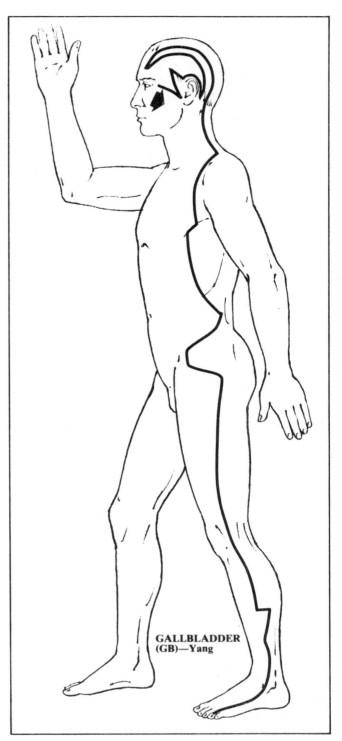

**GALLBLADDER
(GB)—Yang**

8. LIVER – (LV) – Yin

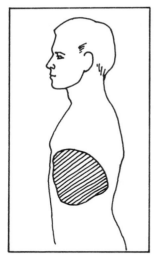

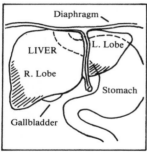

Gallbladder and liver are inseparable organs in both Western and Oriental medicine. Even popular views and expressions in East and West coincide with regard to the liver. When Shakespeare talks about a lily-livered boy in *Macbeth*, he alludes to cowardice. In Greek and Roman times, if the liver of animals sacrificed before battle was blood-red and healthy, it augured well. A pale liver signified defeat. The familiar expression, "He has guts!" reads in Japanese: "He has a strong liver!"

The liver is the largest organ in the human body. It weighs a little more than 3 pounds and is tucked away on the spinal side of the abdominal cavity between stomach and lungs, with most of its mass on the upper right hand side.

The liver is a multi-function gland and performs several *hundred* jobs. Beyond producing bile (see GB), it manufactures and stores vitamin A, it manufactures and stores the agents that clot blood as well as those that prevent clotting, it produces urea and converts glucose to glycogen for storage, then converts it again to glucose when the body needs sugar, it renders toxic substances harmless (modern prescription drugs, for example) and contains cells that remove foreign material from blood. The liver acts as a blood reservoir and produces red blood cells during embryologic development. It is involved in protein and fat metabolism. It generates bicarbonate, which is used to neutralize the Hydrochloric Acid that enters the small intestine from the stomach. It is a magnificent chemical factory. Any malfunctioning produces physical and psychological effects throughout the body. (The abbreviation, LV, has been chosen to avoid confusion with LI, the Large Intestine meridian.)

Location The meridian associated with this vital organ begins near the nail of the big toe and follows a course over the highest portion of the foot and up the inside of the leg and thigh, across the groin area and up to the free end of the eleventh rib.

Function Similar to all the other meridians, working on LV affects a host of symptoms beyond normalizing and balancing the flow of energy along its path and correcting minor liver dysfunctions. Like the liver itself, LV is most notable for its broad effect on soma and psyche, the overall metabolism and mood of the body. It should always be treated when the receiver is recovering from a major disease and when persistent general fatigue signals that all is not well. Note that treating LV helps prevent seasickness.

Treatment LV is best treated with the receiver lying on his back. Use the free hand to support the leg as you apply pressure on the inside.

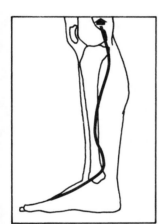

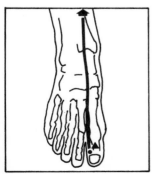

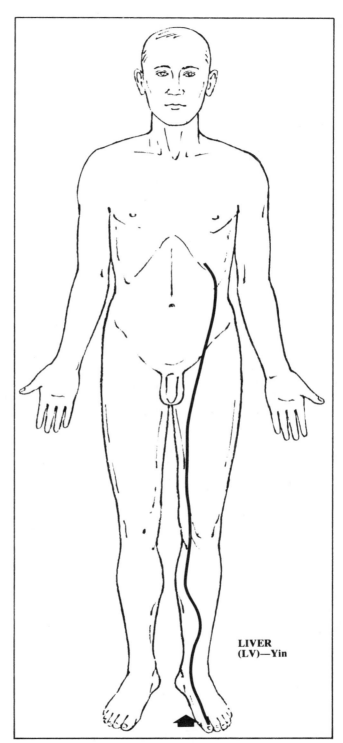

LIVER
(LV)—Yin

33

9. LUNG – (LU) – Yin

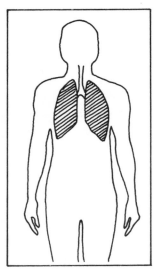

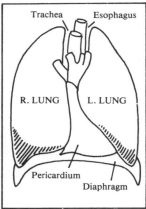

Trachea   Esophagus

R. LUNG   L. LUNG

Pericardium

Diaphragm

The Lung meridian (LU) begins the final cycle of energy. The lungs in Western medicine are specific organs within the respiratory system. Their function is to provide a large epithelial surface for the exchange of oxygen and carbon dioxide. This surface can be as large as 1200 square feet, or the floor space of a family home. Since it is so large, we can live comfortably with only one functioning lung if that should become necessary.

The Oriental conception of lung is significantly wider and includes the entire respiratory tract. The lungs here are seen as the vital organ where CHI, the all-embracing energy of life, enters the body. Lack of CHI leads to general fatigue and reduces the effectiveness of the overall immune system, which in turn makes the body susceptible to nasal congestion, prolonged colds, bronchitis and inflammation in the respiratory tract.

Healthy lungs provide an abundance of CHI—one of the reasons why most Yoga systems place special emphasis on proper breathing, and why some modern Japanese texts on Shiatsu place the Lung meridian (LU) at the beginning of the energy cycle. (See also *The Secret of the Golden Flower, A Chinese Book of Life*, translated and explained by Richard Wilhelm, with a commentary by C.G. Jung. New York: Harcourt, Brace & World).

Location   LU is a Yin meridian. It begins in the hollow area about three fingerbreadths below the outside end of the clavicles, rises a little and then follows a course down the inside of upper arm and forearm. It ends near the base of the thumb nail.

Function   Apart from normalizing and balancing the energy flow in the entire respiratory tract, LU is important for treatment of congestion in all vessels. Point massage along thumb and wrist tends to relieve painful symptoms associated with throat diseases and ear infections.

Treatment   Both LU and its YANG companion, LI, can easily be reached when the receiver is lying down.

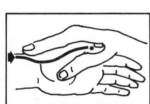

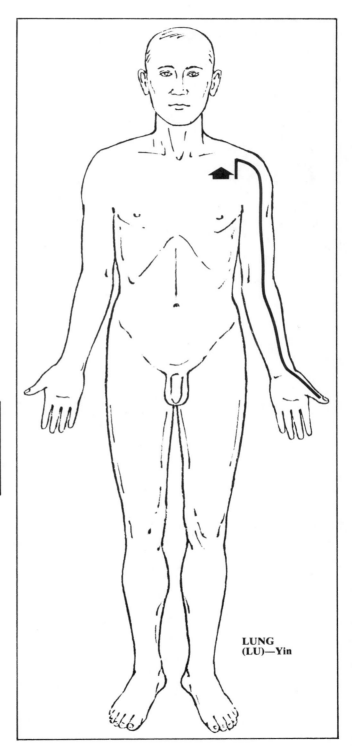

LUNG
(LU)—Yin

10. LARGE INTESTINE – (LI) – Yang

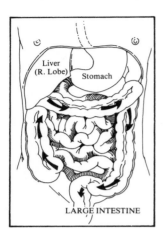

The large intestine is part of the digestive system and connects small intestine and anus. The organ is about five feet long and has a greater diameter than the small intestine. This is where feces are formed when the large intestine absorbs fluid from the waste that reaches it from the small intestine. Diarrhea results when the residue does not remain long enough in the large intestine.

Like the lung, the large intestine is an organ of cleansing and elimination of substances—carbon dioxide from the lungs, digestive residue from the large intestine. Malfunction of the large intestine leads to constipation and, in the Oriental sense, to stagnation of CHI. Like the small intestine, the large intestine requires mucus for lubrication.

Location   The meridian begins on the thumb side of the index finger, near the base of the fingernail, and continues along the wrist. Then it changes course gradually across the forearm and passes the elbow in the manner of a YANG meridian, well on the outside. It continues along the biceps and up to a point on top of the shoulder, moves to the base of the neck, then up past the corner of the mouth. It ends on either side of the nose.

Function   As is usually the case, the meridian is named after the organ it governs, but it must be kept in mind that any organic disturbance or malfunction of a single organ always affects the entire body. It is never an ailing liver that walks into a doctor's office; it is a sick human being. It is never merely a cold and a runny nose; it is aching joints and general fatigue, and the rise in temperature is not restricted to the glowing proboscis alone but can be measured all over.

By the same token, if the major function of an organ is elimination, then the organ does not merely cleanse itself; it purifies the whole body. Treating the LI meridian thus affects detoxification in the body, wherever it occurs. Since the large intestine requires mucus for protection and lubrication, treating LI affects mucous membranes everywhere in the body. The picture in Oriental medicine is always more complex than most Western trained and educated doctors—specialists in particular—are able to see.

Beyond purification and mucus secretion, treating LI improves the metabolism of the body. It is effective against acne and boils; in fact, most skin diseases benefit from regular LI therapy. Strangely, the very beginning of the meridian, the point near the base of the nail of the index finger, affects toothache as well as pain connected with dental work. Next time you see a patient in the dentist's chair pressing his thumb nail into that point while the dentist drills away, rest assured that someone is making good use of the analgesic properties of Shiatsu.

Treatment   For best effect, treat this meridian in combination with its YIN companion, the Lung meridian.

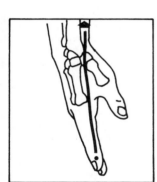

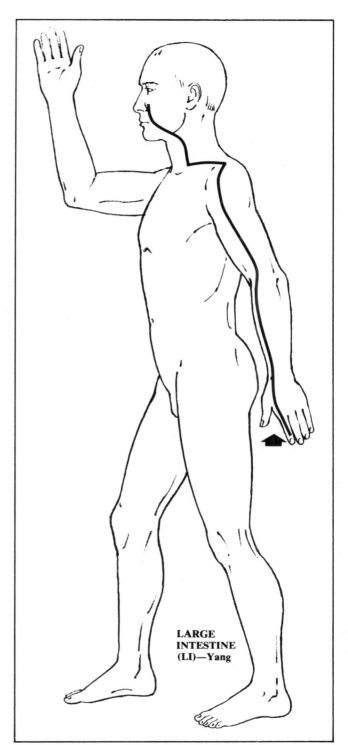

**LARGE
INTESTINE
(LI)—Yang**

11. STOMACH – (ST) – Yang

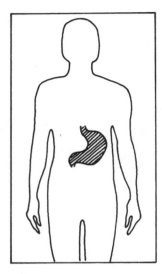

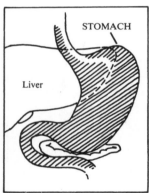

STOMACH

Liver

We chew our food, and when it travels down the esophagus to the stomach, it is called bolus, which is Latin for throw as in throw of dice. Figuratively, bolus also means tidbit. When the food leaves the stomach and moves into the small intestine, it is called chyme, from the Greek word for juice (chymist = chemist).

The stomach is a dilated portion of the digestive tube that connects mouth and anus. Stomachs differ in shape and size with the individual. Their initial function is to store food, which has been reduced in size by the teeth. The next reduction is a chemical one: glands in the stomach wall secrete hydrochloric acid (HCL). This strong acid kills most of the bacteria that have entered with the food and reduces small particles to even smaller ones. HCL has no digestive action on fats and little ability to break down proteins and carbohydrates, but the stomach walls also secrete enzymes (pepsin), which attend to that job. Few nutrients are absorbed by the stomach walls. Most substances are digested later in the small intestine.

The idea of "stomach," in the West and the East, has taken on psychological overtones: we stomach an insult, for example—we swallow it without resentment. Or as in Shakespeare—"He who hath no stomach for this fight" (*Henry V*)—stomach means appetite, but also inclination, and at times wrath. Among the sayings of the Prophet Muhammad we find a thoughtful piece of advice: "The stomach is the home of disease and abstinence the head of every remedy. So make this your custom."

Location The Stomach meridian is YANG and travels from head to toe. It begins in the temporal region and runs past the ear down to the jaw bone, then up to a point below the eye and in line with the pupil. From here it moves to the corner of the mouth, down to the jaw bone again, along the neck to a point near the centre of the clavicles, then outside again and down across the nipples. From here it runs nearly parallel to the Kidney meridian to the groin, then across the knee to the foot, where it ends near the outside corner of the nail on the second toe. The importance of ST is underscored by the fact that Acupuncturists use forty-five tsubos on this meridian.

Function Apart from the obvious—balancing and normalizing the portion of the digestive tract occupied by the stomach—working along ST is also effective against neuralgic facial pains, sores at the corner of the mouth, impotence and frigidity.

Finger pressure on ST along the lower leg reliably alleviates irritability and has a broad effect on hormonal balance, particularly in the genital region. The area immediately below the knee deserves special attention and work here should not be rushed: it restores tranquility and peace of mind.

Treatment For work on both ST and its YIN companion, SP, the receiver is best placed on the carpet.

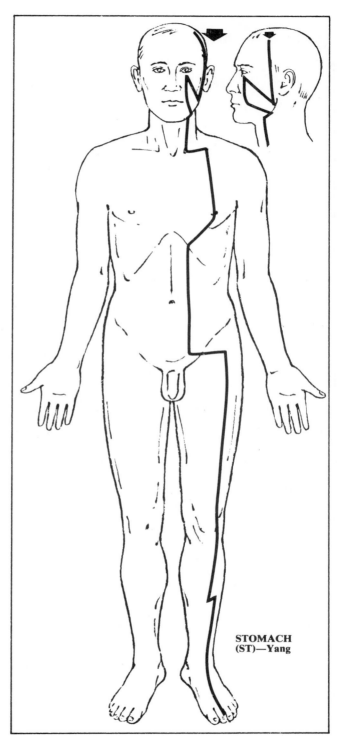

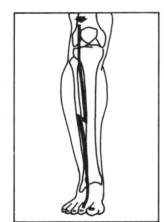

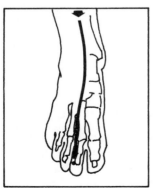

STOMACH (ST)—Yang

12. SPLEEN-PANCREAS - (SP) - Yin

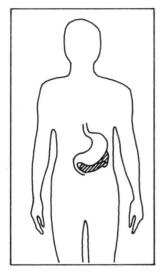

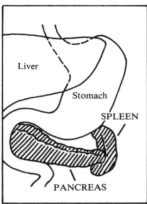

Liver

Stomach

SPLEEN

PANCREAS

In Western medicine, the spleen is part of the lymph-vascular subdivision in the circulatory system. It is located to the left of, and behind, the stomach. Its purpose is to store and filter blood and to remove used-up red blood cells (erythrocytes). The spleen contributes to the body's immune system. It is not considered an essential organ in Western medicine. When it ruptures (accident, sports, especially football), the surgeon will remove it.

In times gone by, when Middle English was spoken, the spleen was regarded as the seat of morose feelings. This meaning is still alive in modern French and German.

Also behind the stomach, and of about the same size as the spleen (5 to 6 inches long), the pancreas can be found. This is an interesting gland that produces and secretes digestive enzymes via the pancreatic duct directly into the duodenum (see SI). These enzymes assist in the digestion of carbohydrates, proteins, fats and nucleic acids. Sodium bicarbonate is also produced here, to neutralize the HCL in the chyme as it comes from the stomach (see ST). Further, at least two hormones are secreted by the pancreas: insulin and glucagon. Insulin stimulates not only the movement of glucose itself, but also the activity of the enzymes that transform the glucose into fat and glycogen. It regulates carbohydrate metabolism and blood sugar levels. The glycogen is stored in the liver and is converted again when the muscles need sugar.

Insulin deficiency, or inadequate response by the body to this hormone, leads to diabetes. Pancreatic diarrhea with large, greasy stools occurs when the digestive enzymes are deficient.

Please keep in mind that Oriental texts mean pancreas, the gland, when they say spleen. Tradition, usage and deference to great practitioners of Oriental medicine have caused the name spleen to be retained. Modern European texts always call the meridian spleen-pancreas (SP).

Location SP is a YIN meridian that begins near the inside base of the big toe nail, moves across the foot and up the leg along the knee cap, then follows the inside edge of the big thigh muscle up to the groin. KI is closest to the centre line of the body, ST is next, and SP is the most lateral meridian on the abdomen. It follows a course to a point near the upper edge of the pectoral muscles and from there drops to its end point on the side of the trunk.

Function Treatment of SP is an excellent way to help overcome daytime sleepiness and fatigue brought about by mental unrest and too much thinking. It stimulates circulation in hands and feet and soothes abdominal spasms. In addition and of equal importance, treating SP normalizes weaknesses in the connective tissue which may show up as cellulitis. Varicose veins and haemorrhoids also benefit, as well as diseases of the female reproductive system, in particular menstrual disorders. It goes without saying that regular SP therapy tends to normalize any pancreatic dysfunction.

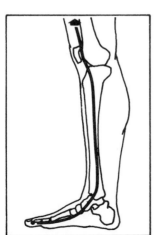

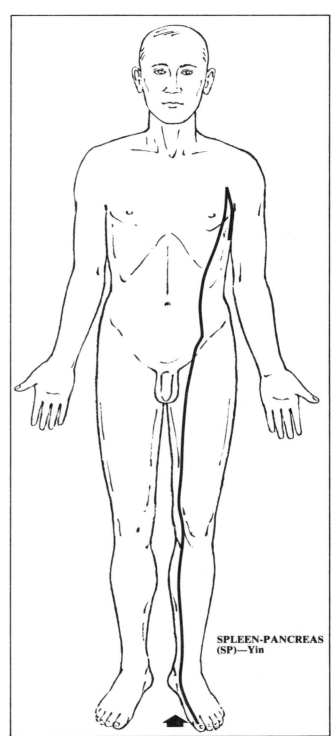

**SPLEEN-PANCREAS
(SP)—Yin**

This concludes the introduction to the twelve major meridians. The cycle is now complete. As the energy rises in SP, it is transferred to the Heart meridian along the trunk and a new cycle begins in the never-ending dance of YIN and YANG.

In addition to the twelve meridians mentioned, Oriental medicine uses eight further meridians. Six of these special meridians establish connections between the twelve meridians already mentioned and use parts of the pathways you already know. The remaining two meridians deserve our special attention. They are extraordinary in that they stand alone and exist as single entities, unlike the twelve major meridians, which always come in mirror-image pairs and have a YIN or YANG partner. To distinguish them further, they are called vessels rather than meridians.

13. CONCEPTION VESSEL – (CV)

This pathway begins in front of the anus and the energy rises across the genitals and the abdomen, sternum and neck to a point above the chin. Anatomically speaking, the vessel covers the ventral median (Latin: venter, stomach). As the name suggests, treatment of CV deals with problems connected with conception, pregnancy and fertility in women and the reproductive organs in men, impotence, for example, or early ejaculation.

Shiatsu in the lower portion of CV between anus and navel connects with the lower Triple Heater and enhances the effectiveness of TH against problems in the urogenital tract. The part between navel and sternum assists the digestive aspect of TH and helps alleviate heartburn, upset stomach and fatigue brought on by too much stress. The upper part normalizes respiratory problems, again in co-operation with TH. As a general rule we can say that health problems on the ventral side of the body benefit from the harmonizing effect of Shiatsu on CV.

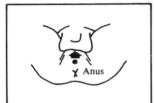

Anus

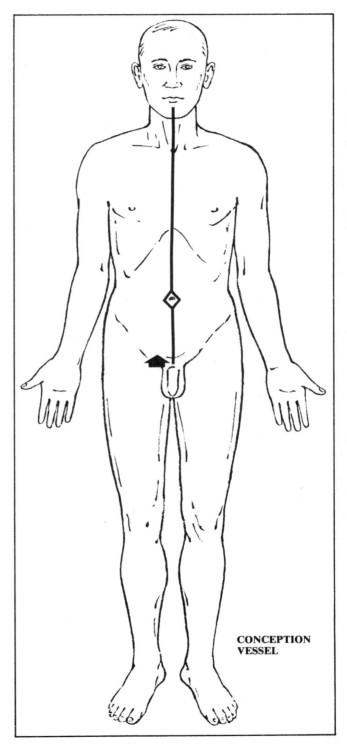

CONCEPTION VESSEL

43

14. GOVERNOR VESSEL – (GV)

GV starts behind the anus and runs up the back and over the head. It ends on a point behind the upper lip above the two incisors. Its path leads precisely over all the spinal knuckles. Anatomically, this is the linea mediana posterior.

As the name suggests, GV governs YIN and YANG harmony on the back of the body. Shiatsu between tailbone and the eighth thoracic vertebrae alleviates physical problems like lumbago, traumatic pain, sexual dysfunction. Above that point, GV begins to exert a beneficial and calming influence on the psyche and is helpful against restlessness, insomnia and lack of concentration. This effect changes again when the pathway reaches the forehead. Shiatsu here relieves headaches and the symptoms of sinusitis. It also helps clear the nasal passages by reducing the swelling of the mucous membranes.

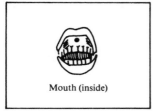

Mouth (inside)

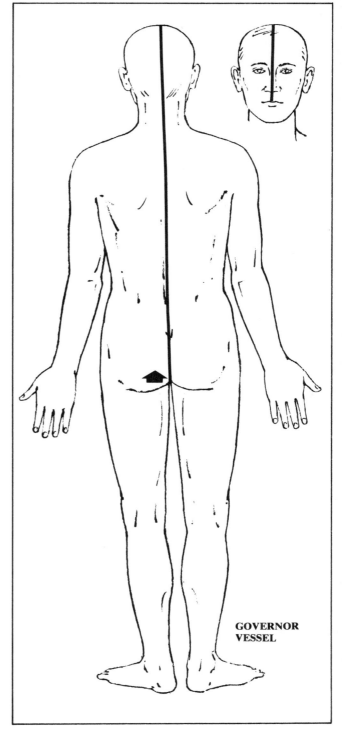

GOVERNOR VESSEL

ON TENSION AND RELAXATION

It is an odd fact that Shiatsu is difficult, if not impossible, to apply to someone who is tense. Those knotted muscles, stiff joints and immobile extremities under your probing fingers do everything to hide the channels of energy and it feels as if there is nothing flowing at all, as if tension has choked the current of life into less than a trickle, as if you were working on a block of marble which by some miracle has attained body temperature. The sensation is not pleasant.

Where does all that tension come from? What do we do about it? Can we avoid it?

First off, life without tension is death. We neither can nor should avoid stress and the tension associated with it. There is no black without white, no YIN without YANG, no relaxation without tension. Things only become dangerous when there is too much of one or the other. Too much relaxation turns us into vegetables. Too much tension and our blood pressure goes up and we lay ourselves open to anything from peptic ulcers to migraine headaches.

Tension arises from stress, which is part of life. Any situation can provoke stress: the raise you didn't get, the driver that cuts in front of you, the evening news, decisions you have to make on the basis of insufficient facts, health, finances, sex—anything at all. Worse than those daily stresses are the ones brought on by unresolved past conflicts. Separation and divorce rank high, but so does the job you somehow slipped into and don't dare let go of now, the relationship that has never really ended, the peer rejection you experienced in grade nine, the feelings of guilt, shame, fear that grew out of one incident or another and were never dealt with. These ghosts from the past form the bottom layer upon which we pile our daily stresses, and we become what disturbs us, because we identify with it.

Unresolved stress eats into your life. It takes away an ever larger portion of CHI and leads to mental fatigue and exhaustion, knotted muscles that haven't been relaxed in years, disturbance that turns into disease and destruction and finally death.

Wanchai Arthavedvoravudhi, one of my teachers, was convinced that cancer, ultimately, is a stress disease. He never let a single lesson go by without reminding us to "Clean out your mental garbage!" Excellent advice. And the earlier in life you start, the easier it is. Eventually you will have to do it anyway. Few of us depart from this life without having reached some manner of peace within ourselves.

METHODS

Of the many relaxation procedures available, I have found that the following one takes care of my students' daily stresses before class:

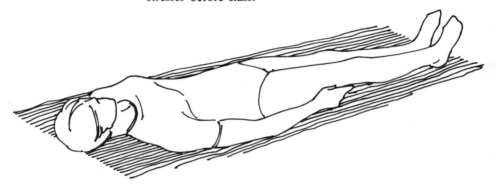

Rest on the carpet, feet slightly apart, hands not touching the body. Close your eyes. Breathe easily and try to relax.

Tense your right fist slowly—nothing else, just your right fist. This involves the muscles of your forearm as well, but no other muscle groups. Be sure of that. Concentrate.

Now relax the fist and feel the slackness in your hand and your forearm.

Sense where the tension went. Did it go up the arm or out through the fingertips? Feel the difference between tension and relaxation. Repeat this several times, always holding the tension for a few heart beats, and then letting go. Now do this with your left fist and repeat. Then with both fists. Tension...and slackness.

Bend your elbows (one at a time) and tighten your biceps. Make them as hard as you can, then relax and straighten out your arm. Repeat this and then do both arms at the same time. Involve as few muscle groups as you are capable of controlling. You will surprise yourself as you find out that this is not as difficult as it sounds. Tighten up—and relax.

Next, tighten up the muscles around your neck, the ones that support your head all day—then relax and feel the difference between the two states. Let deep, warm relaxation sink in. Enjoy it. Then tense up again—and let go.

Where did you send all that tension?

Do the same thing with your head: wrinkle your forehead as much as you can—then smooth it out. Frown and feel the tension spread—then let go. Squint—then relax your eyes. Do the same thing with your jaw, your mouth, your lips. Press your tongue forcefully against the roof of your mouth—and relax your tongue and jaw.

Do the same thing with your shoulders by bringing them up to your ears in a big shrug—then relax and let warmth spread throughout your body.

Fill your lungs and hold your breath tightly—then blow the tension away as you exhale. It helps to imagine a burning candle: blow your tension into the flame and let it burn up. All of it. Next, tighten your stomach muscles, then ease up. Repeat this. Then arch your back and feel the muscles on either side of your spine go taut—and let go.

Tighten the muscles in your buttocks and thighs. You will be surprised how many people hide their daily stresses in that region. (Very descriptive English word, "tight-assed"!) Now, relax and let go. Repeat every exercise at least twice.

Press your heels against the carpet and tense your thighs.

Let go slowly and feel the difference. Study the way relaxation seeps into every muscle. Take your time. Feel your body grow heavier, warmer, as you tense and relax knees, shins, calves, ankles and feet.

Finally, there will be no tension left anywhere in your body. Hold this feeling.

While you are lying there, completely relaxed, turn your thoughts to your partner, who has been doing the same thing. Consider the channels of energy which are now coursing on the surface, easily accessible, ready to be worked on. Think where you will start. Imagine the meridian in your mind—then start.

If you make a tape of this procedure, consider that tensing and relaxing take time. Allow a few moments at each stage to experience the feeling. Initially, twenty minutes of this exercise may only bring partial relaxation. As you become more experienced, a few moments will suffice to take stock of tense muscle groups in your body and it will become an easy habit to direct relaxation into those groups consciously. If you practice yoga, mind-centering and mind-calming techniques will not be strange to you, and the connection between yoga and Shiatsu is obvious and ancient.

Another relaxation technique that works particularly well in small groups is guided imaging. It is exactly what it sounds like: someone creates images in your mind by telling you a simple story. Your guide, for example, takes you on a walk through summer meadows, beside a tall forest, across a shallow brook, to arrive at a safe place. This could be an old cottage in the woods, with a narrow path leading up to it, a trellised gate overgrown with pink roses in full bloom—as you can see, you have already filled in details like the smell of the roses, the murmuring of the brook, the robin on the fence. The group, of course, relaxes on the carpet again, eyes closed, listening.

Two things are important when this technique is employed: there must be no threatening images of any kind, no motorized traffic, for instance. And the safe place must be something anybody can identify with and feel good about. If you lead your group into the snake pit of the nearest zoo, all you will do is create tension.

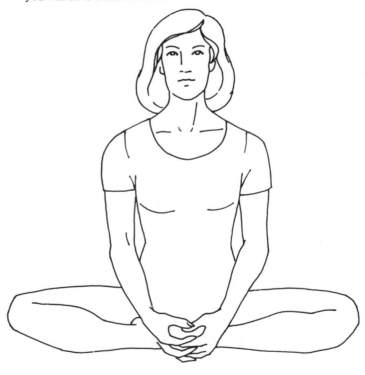

The relaxing benefits of meditation must not be forgotten. The common goal of all meditation is the quieting of that chatterbox, the everyday mind. In Transcendental Meditation, as in some schools of yoga, this is achieved with the help of a mantra, a word/sound, at times without meaning. The

Rinzai school of Zen uses a Koan instead, a riddle without logical solution, to focus the mind (What is the clapping of one hand?). Sufi meditators practice the repetition of a religious formula to attain a meditative state. We in the West are only just beginning to unravel the mysteries of meditation.

A leisurely hot bath relaxes most people. Some practitioners swear by the soothing effect of hot towels, which they place on tense muscle groups. Ideally, the receiver should spend an hour in a flotation tank before a Shiatsu session. There is no more effective method to achieve near total relaxation in so short a time. If you have never floated, find out if there is a Floating Centre in your area and try it. You may get hooked and eventually build your own tank in the basement—a matchless investment for your mental and physical health.

For the purpose of practicing Shiatsu, we can sit quietly for a few minutes and simply meditate on health and well-being, both our own and that of our partner. We can tune in to this other person whose energy field we are about to share. We can clear our minds of troubling thoughts and concentrate on what we are about to do.

Nothing happens in Shiatsu unless both partners are relaxed and aware. A few minutes of quiet thought is the minimum. Find out what works for you, then use it. Repetition creates familiarity. If you find that guided imaging relaxes you, then learn to make the trip without spoken words. The exercise routine may be just what you need; commit the sequence to memory.

Experienced Shiatsu practitioners will go to great lengths in order to create a feeling of warmth and well-being before they begin to work. One Sun, Sunim, always went through an informal tea ceremony and quickly established an atmosphere of serene trust and confidence before class. There is no reason why you and your partner should not do the same. The more relaxed you are, the deeper the effect of Shiatsu will be.

DIAGNOSIS

Here is a list of symptoms: lack of appetite, meteorism, anxiety, diarrhea, chills, nausea, headache, coughing, excessive sweating, bloated feeling. Now, what is the disease that causes all this?

Lack of appetite is caused by gastritis. Cirrhosis of the liver produces wind (meteorism). Angina pectoris is the obvious reason for anxiety, and typhoid fever spawns diarrhea. The chilly feeling is caused by tuberculosis, and there must be appendicitis around somewhere; why else the nausea? Headache points to chronic sinusitis, and pleurisy is the reason for the cough. The thyroid gland works overtime, hence the production of excessive sweat. The bloated feeling points to a serious infection of the duodenum. No doubt the patient will terminate shortly.

While all the diseases cited agree perfectly with the symptoms, another explanation is equally feasible: Harry's birthday party. It lasted all night. The cabbage rolls were flown in from the Ukraine for the occasion, the wine came from Chile and the music was provided by The Blind Dates from Pasadena (dressed in costume). Nobody noticed that the air conditioning failed halfway through the long night and visibility in the crowded place dropped to less than ten feet within minutes.

A good night's sleep, a cold shower and a long walk in fresh air will clear things up. Our patient has miraculously recovered.

DIAGNOSIS ON THE URINARY BLADDER MERIDIAN

Diagnosis is never a simple matter. Years of training come into play when you visit your physician (as you should, regularly). Urine and blood are analyzed, reflexes are checked, and if something seems seriously wrong, one or more specialists will look into it.

If you visit an Acupuncturist in Hong Kong, five thousand years of experience culminate in the way the man feels your pulse on both wrists and with both hands, using three fingers on each side and measuring the intensity of your pulse at different depths. Pulse diagnosis is an integral part of Acupuncture.

You will be surprised at the detailed questions a Homeopathic Physician will ask you before he prescribes anything. Homeopaths have developed anamnesis (the history of a patient's disease) to near perfection. Practitioners of Naturopathic Medicine may use the tongue for diagnosis, or the iris. They may use a modern development of an ancient system—electro-acupuncture diagnosis—or establish the surface temperature distribution of your body and reach conclusions about the current state of health of internal organs from the pattern of infrared radiation.

None of these polished techniques apply within the context of this book. We are after a general state of well-being. Diagnosis on this plane is relatively simple. All we want to know is whether CHI, the universal energy, is flowing freely and unimpeded through all twelve major meridians. If this is the case, then we can be certain that we are in good shape physically and most likely mentally as well. On the other hand, if energy flow has stagnated in some place, we would like to know where, so that we can correct the situation.

UB, the Urinary Bladder meridian, provides us with the necessary diagnostic points. You will recall that this longest meridian runs down your back in two lanes on both sides of the spine. It is the inner lanes, two fingerbreadths away from the spinal ridge on each side, that concern us here. As you can see from the drawing, the diagnostic points are all neatly lined up between shoulders and buttocks.

These points will become sensitive to pressure if energy flow in the associated meridian is disturbed. The problem, then, is to find the precise location of each set of diagnostic points. This is not as difficult as it may sound.

You know that the inner branches of UB are two fingerbreadths distant from the median (use the receiver's fingers for measurement). You also know what a human spine looks like. As long as you can count the knuckles on the spine (the spinous processes) and maintain two fingerbreadths distance, there is no reason why you should not find the points. The first ten pairs are always located in between two vertebrae—eight on the thoracic curve and two on the lumbar curve. The remaining two can be found on the sacrum, the fused portion of the spine between lumbar curve and coccyx (tail bone).

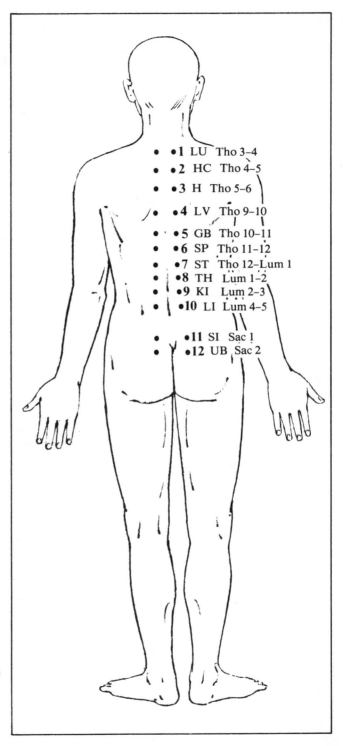

●1 LU Tho 3–4
●2 HC Tho 4–5
●3 H Tho 5–6
●4 LV Tho 9–10
●5 GB Tho 10–11
●6 SP Tho 11–12
●7 ST Tho 12–Lum 1
●8 TH Lum 1–2
●9 KI Lum 2–3
●10 LI Lum 4–5
●11 SI Sac 1
●12 UB Sac 2

**DIAGNOSTIC POINTS
ON THE INNER
BRANCH OF THE
URINARY BLADDER
MERIDIAN**

At the base of the neck there is one prominent bone protruding from the spine: the seventh and last cervical vertebra—a good point to start counting from. The next knuckle down is number one on the thoracic curve. The shoulder blades provide another sign post: a line across their lowest points falls across the eighth thoracic vertebra. Lastly, a line across the narrowest part of the waist runs between the second and third vertebrae on the lumbar curve. The lumbar curve has only five vertebrae and their spinous processes are easily counted.

The sacrum is a solid bone comprising five fused sacral vertebrae. The diagnostic points for SI are located on either side of the first spinous process on the sacrum. Finally, the diagnostic points for UB, the Urinary Bladder meridian itself, are located two fingerbreadths from either side of the second spinous process on the sacrum.

If you can learn to find these twenty-four points on your partner's back, you have mastered a very basic system of diagnosis. No more is required on this level. There are dozens of other points on the human body that will assist, confirm, narrow down and cross-check, but at this time they do not concern us and would only serve to confuse.

PROCEDURE

If you press point eight between the first and second lumbar vertebrae with your thumb or index finger, and you find a spot that is painful, less elastic than the surrounding skin, a little hard, then something is wrong with the energy flow in TH, the Triple Heater meridian. It doesn't tell you more. Inasmuch as TH is concerned with respiration, digestion and the urogenital tract, the disturbance could be in one, two, or all three areas. If your partner shows no symptoms and nothing is obviously wrong, then treat it as a warning sign: you have caught a disturbance well before it shows up as a disease. You are working in the area where Shiatsu functions best.

To remedy the situation, treat both TH and its companion, the Heart Constrictor meridian, HC. Some of the psychic and emotional overtones from one meridian inevitably spill over into its YIN-YANG partner, so it is always best to treat one YIN-YANG pair during the same session.

If you detect a painful spot between the third and the fourth thoracic vertebrae, the disturbance sits in the Lung meridian, LU. In that case, both LU and LI should be treated. The therapeutic procedure is covered in the next chapter.

DIAGNOSTIC POINTS ON THE VERTEBRAE

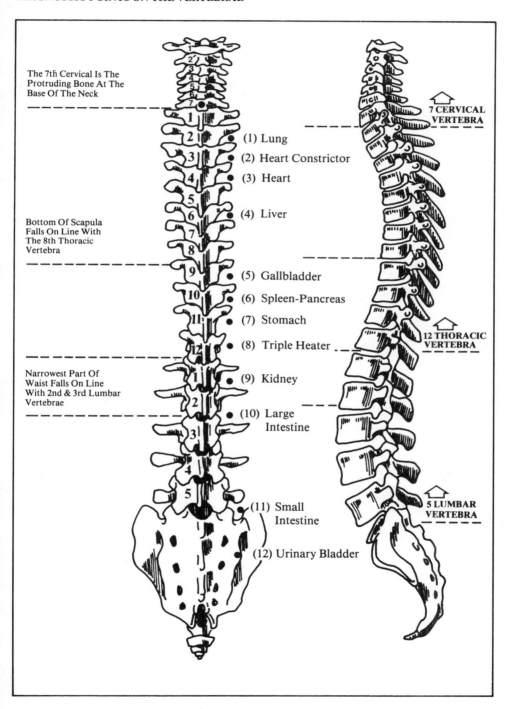

The 7th Cervical Is The Protruding Bone At The Base Of The Neck

Bottom Of Scapula Falls On Line With The 8th Thoracic Vertebra

Narrowest Part Of Waist Falls On Line With 2nd & 3rd Lumbar Vertebrae

(1) Lung

(2) Heart Constrictor

(3) Heart

(4) Liver

(5) Gallbladder

(6) Spleen-Pancreas

(7) Stomach

(8) Triple Heater

(9) Kidney

(10) Large Intestine

(11) Small Intestine

(12) Urinary Bladder

7 CERVICAL VERTEBRA

12 THORACIC VERTEBRA

5 LUMBAR VERTEBRA

THE COMPLETE TREATMENT

PREPARATION

Preparation is half the battle. During a treatment, consult the drawings in the book only if you absolutely have to—it is very disturbing to divide your attention between a page and your fingers. Time spent committing the meridians to memory is an excellent investment.

The pathways of energy on the surface of the human body can be learned in many ways. Retention of images is so well developed in some people that all they have to do is stare at the drawing for a time, and they have it. This is rare. Most people learn by doing. Perfection comes with regular practice.

My classroom students start out by working on each other. Meridians are first introduced through slides and drawings. They are discussed and redrawn, if necessary. Some students do their homework with body paint during the initial learning phase, carefully transferring meridians from page to skin. (Marker pens are not recommended.) Before a treatment, partners consider the meridians to be treated, where they are and what they do, and discuss them.

Once you start a treatment, you must try to picture the meridian to be explored. You are trying to fix a channel in your mind. Concentrate on the path of energy and memorize what your finger tells you about skin, bones and muscles. Sense what your hand tells you about tension in the arm you are holding. Recognize landmarks along the path, hard spots, soft spots, muscles and tendons. Treat the meridian on the other side of the body, noting the subtle differences between left and right. It is better to complete a treatment smoothly and not break the rhythm, even if you miss the path here and there. You will do better on the next run.

BREATHING AND MASSAGE

When you begin to investigate the diagnostic points along UB on your partner's back, you will become conscious of his breathing rhythm as your fingers rise and fall. Please pay special attention to this pattern.

Unlike our heartbeat, over which we have no direct control, we can influence the way we exhale and inhale. We can hold our breath consciously—and we can forget about it altogether, in which case the body takes over and respiration happens automatically, as it does most of the time. Breathing thus offers us a unique way of entering into deliberate control of one vital bodily function. Once breathing is mastered, we may achieve conscious control over other bodily functions as well and thus raise our level of awareness. This is the way of YOGA. The word means union, in the sense of uniting the individual with a higher reality. Simply put, we learn to see more because we become more aware of all realities, including our own.

In its finest form, Shiatsu achieves the same thing by using the same open door: your partner's breathing pattern. It provides you with the basic slow and calm rhythm of the entire treatment. By adopting this pattern to the way you trace the meridians and apply pressure, you and your partner become one healing unit. All sense of "I do this..." slowly fades away as the rhythm takes over and both giver and receiver become subordinate to the breathing pattern. The effect is quite extraordinary and overwhelming when it happens for the first time. It is love, but not of the romantic kind.

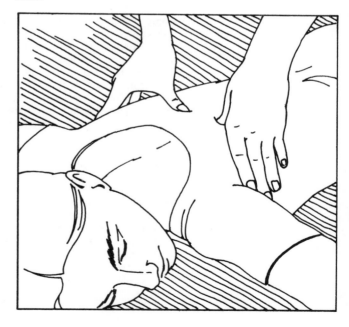

As your partner exhales and the thorax contracts, you follow this movement down with your thumbs, pushing slightly. At the lowest point, you hold the position of your thumbs and wait for inhalation to begin. There is always a pause. Then you let your partner push against your thumbs as he inhales. This may be painful. Adjust the pressure until the pain feels good, hold it for a few heartbeats, then move your thumbs up and slide along the meridian about 2 inches to the next position. At exhalation, follow the movement of the thorax down to the lowest point again and hold, wait for the thumbs to be pushed up again, slide to the next position and continue to follow the pattern.

Once you become aware of this rhythm, the way a fisherman is aware of the state of the tide at any time of day or night without having to stop and think about it, then you are on the right track. Treating UB first makes it particularly easy to slip into this tidal rhythm. You can do it with your eyes closed, and then continue in the same beat as you move off the thoracic and into the lumbar and sacral regions. If you stop to massage a sensitive point along the way, pick up the rhythm again when you continue, always pressing with exhalation and moving (after a slight delay) to the next position as your partner inhales.

A word about pain feeling good: remember when, in grade two, you began to lose your baby teeth? How you spent hours pushing with tongue and tooth against a wiggling canine or a premolar that was just about ready to come out, but not quite? Sure, it was painful, yet it was more a kind of pleasure-pain, bearable, tempting, difficult to leave alone. It is exactly this kind of pain we are after when we slide our thumbs along the meridians and press. To tell you that 7½ pounds of pressure is roughly right would be misleading. Everybody has a slightly different pain threshold. Let your partner be your guide. Very little pressure is required on the head, a little more along the meridians on the ventral side, and much more on back and legs.

Of course, any heroics are completely misplaced. This is not a contest to find out how much pressure you can stand or how much pain you can inflict. (If the Marquis de Sade ever heard about Shiatsu, it doesn't show up in his writing.) Some well-muscled males require the point of your elbow and the weight of your body on their trapezius muscles, because the thumb will simply not get through. With children, the point of the index finger is quite enough.

CONTACT

Always use one hand to hold and support the limb you are working on. This will establish another habit: never lose contact with your partner during Shiatsu therapy. Later, as you begin working on UB for example, you will find yourself moving around from head to toe and from one side to the other. As you do this, keep one hand on your partner at all times. This lets him know where you are and the next touch

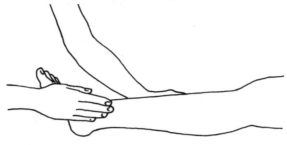

of your thumb does not come unexpectedly—which, at best, is somewhat unsettling, and at worst upsets the whole pattern of treatment. On a deeper level, keeping one hand on your receiver at all times is reassuring. Nobody likes to feel alone and abandoned. Well-trained massage therapists know this.

PRESSUSRE POINTS (TSUBOS)

When you come across a sensitive point on your travels along a meridian, take a little time to massage the point gently until the pain disappears.

Think of these points as railroad switches. As long as the system is functioning as it should, the well-oiled switches move of their own accord and divert the trains of energy to where they do the most good, preventing here an overload and there depletion and lack. Once the system is disturbed (X-rays will do that too, for example), the switches are no longer functioning as they should. They have become rusty—sensitive to pressure.

If you trace the meridians carefully, in time you will learn to distinguish between meridian and tsubo. Your finger tips will become so educated that they recognize the distinct feel of a tsubo, a slight difference in temperature, a hardness that feels like an impossibly small muscle knot, a mushroom the size of a pinhead pushing up. Getting to know the diagnostic points along UB is of great help, because you can pinpoint them with more precision than most other tsubos and thus learn how they feel different.

TREATMENT

We start treatment with the UB-KI cycle, because we are interested in what the diagnostic points have to tell us. Another reason for always starting with UB-KI has to do with our Western way of eating. We can no longer avoid ingesting minute amounts of toxic substances every day. We eat on the run and we drink even when we are not thirsty. The air we breathe is no longer clean and pure, and the toxins we inhale enter the blood stream through the lungs. UB and KI are both concerned with elimination and cleansing. Starting a Shiatsu treatment with the UB-KI cycle begins a detoxification program in the body that purifies without forcing you to go on a fast. You encourage the body under your hands to get rid of poisons, which have become one of the major factors in the phenomenal growth of chronic diseases today.

Purification has become vital. If you have time for nothing else, then do at least UB and KI, and you have done well.

Find a time when you can take the phone off the hook for a couple of hours. No television. No radio. No alcohol or drugs. Your fingernails are short. The room is warm. Wear loose clothing—T-shirt and shorts in the summer, jogging suit in the winter time. You have made a tape of the relaxation procedure and spent a half hour on the carpet listening to his voice, or yours, guiding you through various muscle groups, tensing and relaxing, conscious of every finger, every toe and every breath—until the great warmth of relaxation has enveloped you both and you are ready to begin.

Your partner sits up—on the floor or on a low chair (a Za-Zen bench is ideal)—and you kneel behind him and place your hands lightly on his shoulders on either side of, and close to, the neck. Under your palms are now SI and TH as well as GB. Under your fingers are LI, LU, SP and

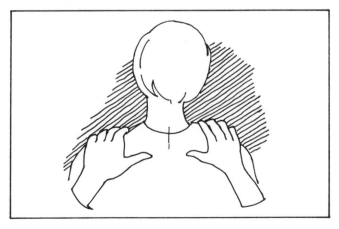

ST—seven meridians. Knowing this, it will not surprise you that most people hide their tension in the big multi-function trapezius muscle.

Close your eyes and do nothing for a moment. Take a while to intuit which of the two sides under your hands is stronger. Do not mistake remnants of tension (hardness) for strength.

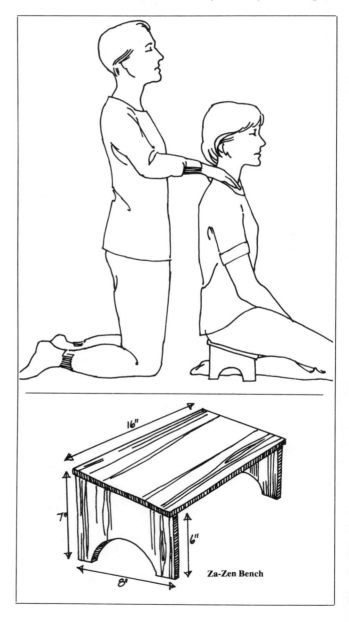

Za-Zen Bench

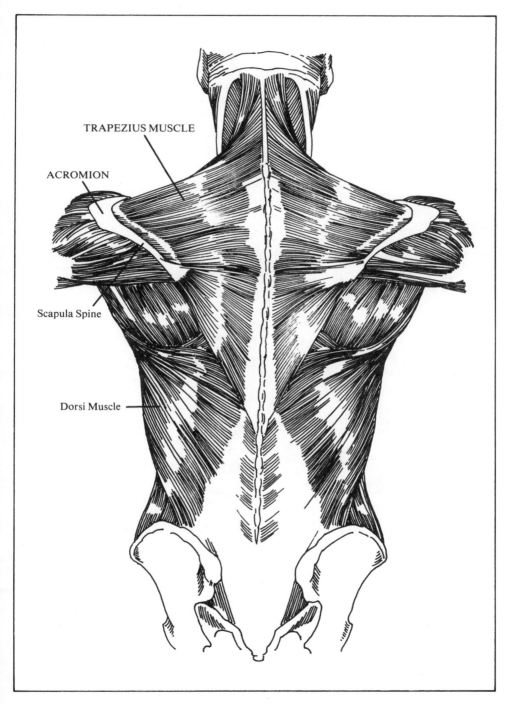

TRAPEZIUS MUSCLE

ACROMION

Scapula Spine

Dorsi Muscle

What you want to sense is vitality, life, energy flow, CHI in the seven meridians under your hands. Let the decision come to you, then start with the stronger side and gently knead the trapezius muscle until it becomes pliant like dough, while the other hand rests on the weaker side, doing nothing. From now on, there will always be at least one hand on your partner's body until the treatment is complete.

Next, do the same thing to the other side until both shoulders feel evenly supple. Now slide both hands down the upper arms to the elbows, grab biceps and triceps with the force of a modest handshake, release the pressure, slide upwards an inch, press, release and slide upwards again. Do

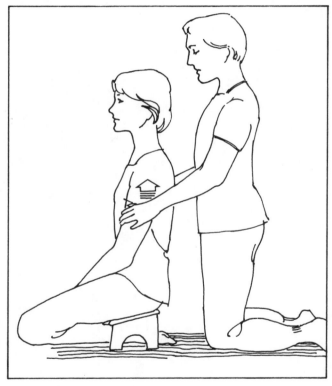

this rapidly until you have reached the base of the neck, then slide your hands down slowly again and repeat a few times. It will drive away the remaining hidden tension in the area. When both shoulders feel perfectly relaxed, use your thumbs and slide them from the acromion along the upper ridge of the trapezius muscle. After they have covered one-third the distance, press both thumbs simultaneously into the upper ridge and hold the pressure for a few heartbeats, release and press again when you have reached the second third. Finally, knead the upper shoulder area again and then slide your hands gently down to the elbows several times. This is exactly what it seems to be: a caress. You are telling the body under your fingers that you mean it no harm. You evoke trust. You are breaking through an old and distressing Western taboo against touching another human being.

When the shoulders are relaxed, use one hand to support the head of your partner, and with the index finger of the other hand begin tracing UB on the opposite side.

Press the starting point near the root of the nose—release and slide upwards—press above the eyebrow—release and slide to the centre of the forehead just below the hair line—press, then release and slide along the scalp.

Work this way until you have reached a point in the hollow near the hair line on the back of the skull, then do the other branch of UB on the head the same way, ending on the other side of the hollow at the base of the skull. Always support the head on the side opposite to where you slide and press.

Now help your partner lie face down on the carpet. Remember: never lose touch! Make sure his head is comfortable and his arms are stretched out along his body. Take the back of his right foot into your left hand, and the back of his left foot into your right (not the soles: the back!). This way, they are crossed over. Using your weight and not your strength, push the heels toward the buttocks slowly, hold for a few heartbeats, then move them towards you, recross the feet and do it again. Use one hand for each foot and do not press with one foot against the other. Let your hands and your weight do the pressing. Then lay the feet down again.

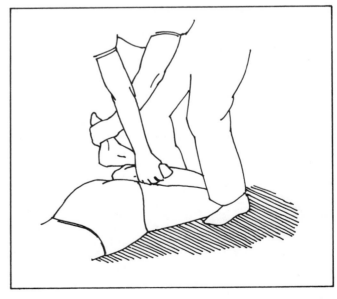

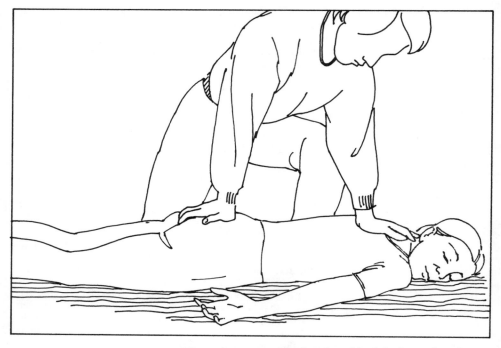

Next, place your right hand on his right buttock and your left hand on his left shoulder blade, then bend over him and put all your weight into your hands. This stretches your partner crosswise. Hold that pressure for a moment, release slowly, slide your hands over to the left buttock/right shoulder blade and repeat. It is best to do this with elbows locked. That way you are forced to use your weight and let gravity work for you, rather than use your strength. Now you are ready to work on the inner branch of the Urinary Bladder meridian, UB.

Straddle your partner (don't sit on him!), or you can kneel to either side on one knee, whichever is more convenient for you, and work with elbows locked, using your thumbs. Starting at the base of the skull, trace the left and right branches of UB simultaneously with your thumbs, sliding for about two inches, pressing, then sliding again.

Start counting from the seventh cervical vertebra (the prominent bone at the base of the neck), and check LU between Tho 3–4. If there is any pain, your partner will tell you. In order for this to work, it is important that you not vary the pressure. Be consistent throughout back and legs. Use less pressure on head and abdomen and, again, be consistent. It is easy to cause pain by simply increasing pressure, but if you do, you miss the point of the exercise, if you'll pardon the pun.

If the LU tsubos are unduly sensitive, make a mental note and gently massage them for a few moments before continuing. This massage is best done with your index finger: place it on the point, note how it feels different from the rest of the meridian, then slide your index finger slowly clockwise (stimulation) or counter-clockwise (sedation). Ask your partner which motion feels better.

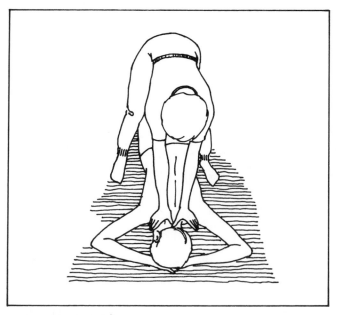

Next, check HC between Tho 4–5, then H between Tho 5–6, and so on, until you reach the UB point on top of the buttocks. Sedate or stimulate sensitive points in accordance with your partner's wishes.

You may find that not a single point is more sensitive to pressure than the rest of the meridian: congratulations! All is as it should be. On the other hand, if several points prove painful, make a mental note of the most sensitive one. The most sensitive point is the one whose meridian and YIN-YANG partner you will treat after you have done the UB-KI cycle. In time you will do this quite automatically.

To continue, follow UB on both legs simultaneously down to the knee, always sliding your thumbs approximately two inches, then pressing. From the knee on it is better to treat each lower leg separately. This is best done by supporting the back of each foot on your thigh—the curves fit nicely into each other, and the calf muscles remain relaxed, so the meridian is easy to find.

Walk your hands up your partner's back (never lose touch!), and start the second branch of UB, again simultaneously on both sides of the spine, using your thumbs and kneeling alongside or straddling your partner. Follow it through right down to the little toe again, treating each lower leg separately. The lower legs thus get treated twice.

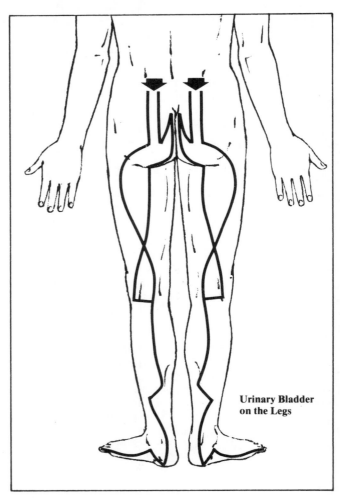

Urinary Bladder on the Legs

Help your partner turn over on his back and begin KI between the balls of the big and little toes under the foot. Treat each leg separately up to the groin area. KI is a YIN meridian and runs along the inside of the leg, so use your free hand to support the outside of the leg as you trace-push-trace-push up the inside. From the groin, the meridian runs one fingerbreadth from either side of the centre line on the abdomen. Use your index finger here. Less pressure is required because the muscles and underlying tissue are softer.

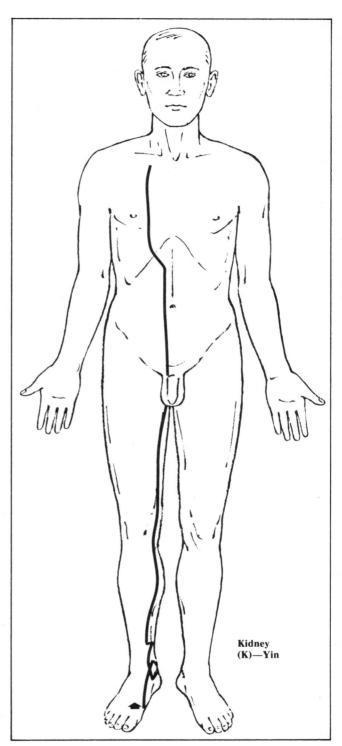

Kidney
(K)—Yin

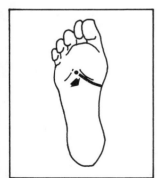

With KI completed, you now turn your attention to the meridian associated with the most painful diagnostic point. If this happens to be LU, then treat LU and its partner, LI. If it happens to be SP, then ST should be treated as well.

Always use the same procedure. That is, press the starting point of the meridian, slide along it for approximately two inches, using little pressure, then press again. Any sensitive points you encounter along the way should be massaged until the pain fades.

The whole treatment in a nut shell:

Establish a calm setting
Do a relaxation exercise together
Relax the shoulders and upper arms
Begin treatment with UB on the head
Continue treatment of UB on the back
Note sensitive diagnostic points
Complete UB
Turn your partner over
Finish basic treatment with KI
Treat the meridian associated with a painful diagnostic spot
Treat its YIN-YANG partner
Rest
Finally, check the painful diagnostic spot on the inner branch of UB again: chances are, the pain has lessened or the point has vanished altogether.

Every once in a while it happens that the receiver simply falls asleep during treatment. Fatigue has taken over or you have carried out the relaxation exercise particularly well. In that case, stop working and cover your partner with a blanket. For that session you have done all you can.

One Shiatsu session with relaxation exercise, UB, KI and two more meridians takes about 2 hours. I would suggest that for the first three months you have one session a week in order to get the detoxification program started. Alternate from week to week between giver and receiver.

RESULTS

Initially, your specific condition may worsen for a week or two. This situation will pass quickly, though. There is no cause for alarm. In fact, it is quite common and normal in most non-poisonous and non-destructive therapies. Channels that have been dry and dormant for years are suddenly urged to perform again, and for a time you will find painful tsubos in the most unexpected places. Years of living have caused every organ in your body to deteriorate to a certain degree. Repair work takes time. Do not expect to regain perfect, glowing health in two Shiatsu sessions if it took you fifteen years or more to reach your current state.

After three months of regular Shiatsu, general improvement will begin to show up and you will look forward to the time set aside for the session. Awareness and sensitivity have increased and you are making discoveries now—about yourself as well as your partner. Things happen. You may actually see a meridian run as a slight discoloration (most often dark pink) a few inches ahead of the point where your thumbs are working: all you have to do is follow the line.

At about this time you will also know precisely where the meridians are located on this person you are working with. You will no longer detect tsubos entirely by accident. Your fingers will recognize them along the paths and will expect to find them in specific places, like old friends waiting patiently to be hugged.

Little by little, the pattern under your hands is changing now, and a tsubo that was painful last week has disappeared—a good sign that things are beginning to work. Other tsubos will show up as the beneficial influence of your fingers makes itself felt throughout the body. There is no need to map them: your fingers will remember every single one as you get to know this human being in a new way—your partner, an entity of energy.

Sometimes when working on a meridian, a streak of warmth will seem to radiate the full length of the pathway. This means that you have cleared up an old blockage. It also serves to explain why treating the lower leg may suddenly relieve a stubborn headache: symptoms are not always situated close to where the disturbance has occurred. Energy surges through the entire body. A blockage on the scalp may alleviate pain in an aching joint. This is why it is important to treat both meridians of a YIN-YANG cycle at one time, because a rusty switch in one affects the other as well.

Something else will happen, too: you will for long moments now stop living in your head alone. Your fingers will become extensions of your body, rather than of your intellect. You will find them moving along the meridians as if drawn by invisible strings, guided by your inner compass. You will discover the many minute deviations of individual meridians from the chart—which can never give more than a very close approximation of courses, channels and pathways. Your partner is not a piece of parchment. He is as unique and singular as you yourself are. Trust this intuition as it develops. Your body knows what it is doing. Don't override your fingers with intellectual commands if you find them tracing a path half-an-inch away from where the chart says it should be.

In time you will treat friends, and things will be different again. You will intuit the same energies coursing along their paths, but neither will the tracks be exactly the same, nor will the distribution of energy match that of your first partner. Exploration and discovery begin anew and you will learn through direct experience, body to body, rather than through "information" handed down in print, via television or through chalk-and-talk. Touch it—and you will learn. You will accept what is, rather than look for what ought to be.

It all starts with getting to know one human being intimately on a level completely different from what you have experienced before. This takes time. Be patient.

AND FINALLY

In spite of its venerable age, Chinese medicine is neither timeworn, nor has it faded in importance. Research is progressing on many fronts, and attempts at combining Western medicine with the traditional Chinese system look promising (especially at the medical faculty of Tongji University in Wuhan, Hupeh Province, in the People's Republic of China).

Beginning to learn Shiatsu has introduced you to the essential difference between the two approaches: Western medicine tries to identify a disease, and then fight it. Chinese medicine is more concerned with the entire spectrum of symptoms and strives to restore overall health. Western medicine frequently puts up with a host of side effects and complications which are rarely ever caused by Chinese therapies.

Shiatsu can be the beginning of a transformational journey. By far the biggest obstacle in this process is the regularity, persistence, the sameness of a simple routine carried out week after week, the predictability of a pattern. Yet a Chinese Tai-Chi practitioner finds nothing unusual or strenuous about the voluntary daily repetition of 175 movements, of refining them over many years until they can be performed in a smooth sequence. For most Westerners, such a routine calls for some mental re-programming.

Some of my students have found it helpful to organize in a small group that meets once a week to continue the work on meridional therapy. That way they feel obliged to attend, and regular therapy develops into a habit. The relaxation exercise more often than not becomes a serene tea ceremony. Three couples appears to be the most successful and lasting combination.

With regular practice, the material presented in this book can be mastered in about a year. Where do you go from there? Nowhere, I hope. You and your partner can not be healthier than healthy. Superhealth is a modern myth. You have achieved normality—your own normality, which should not be confused with average health. If average health were the norm, then chronic intestinal infection, decayed teeth and permanent postural damage would describe a healthy human being. To a Shiatsu practitioner, this is not acceptable.

Transformation to normality and excellent health will be so gradual that your friends will notice the changes much earlier than you will. You are still the same person, doing the same job, splitting firewood and carrying water. Awareness of energetic patterns will not dawn upon you like some overwhelming cataclysmic event. Calm and patience are required to sense the minute tremors that indicate ongoing change and improvement in your partner and yourself. Looking back after a few years, you will marvel at the simplicity of the system and wonder how you ever did without it.

FURTHER READING

Like many Shiatsu practitioners, I have over the years accumulated an extensive reference library on the subject of meridional therapy. Yet I find it difficult to recommend any single book on the subject.

There is a deluge of recent publications on Shiatsu available from Japan. No doubt most of them were written with great sincerity, and some have grown from years of practical experience. But it must be difficult to find translators who are equally at home, not only in both languages, but also in the various fields of medicine, particularly anatomy and physiology. Howlers are unavoidable.

On the serious side, I have found some of the drawings downright wrong. When a popular Japanese text (selling in Canada for $21.95) shows the Stomach meridian running along the *inside* of the lower leg, then obviously the drawings have not been checked for errors, and the book was produced in haste. For a beginner, it is difficult to spot these blunders. For a practitioner, it is painful to see an ancient and effective system abused.

Perhaps the best advice I can give is: go back to the source. Since we are dealing with Acupuncture without needles, any translation of a Chinese text on Acupuncture will broaden your view and deepen your understanding.

The Academy of Oriental Heritage publishes *The Yellow Emperor's Book of Acupuncture*, an excellent translation from the Chinese, by Dr. Henry C. Lu. This is text number 300 of the Chinese Medicine Study Series, available in Canada from P.O. Box 35057, Station "E," Vancouver, BC V6M 4G1, and in the U.S. from P.O. Box 8066, Blaine, WA 98230.

You may find an atlas of meridians and pressure points helpful. The one published by Happiness Press, 160 Wycliff Way, Magalia, CA 95954, is poster-size and authentic.

Much thorough research in the field is being carried out in

Europe, and one of the best current text books is the one by Johannes Bischko, M.D., *Einfuhrung In Die Akupunktur*, also available in English as *An Introduction to Acupuncture* through Karl F. Haug, publishers, Heidelberg.

Beyond that, you are on your own, and the ancient Roman advice is as valid as ever: *caveat emptor*—buyer, beware. A visit to your local library may save you a lot of money and much frustration. Better yet, find a competent teacher in your area.

Among experienced small boat sailors there is a saying: It takes seven years to make a sailmaker, and many more to make a good one. The same applies to Shiatsu practitioners.

INDEX OF SYMPTOMS